Awakening from Alzheimer's

How 9 Maverick Doctors are Reversing Alzheimer's,
Dementia and Memory Loss

By Peggy Sarlin

Awakening from Alzheimer's:

How 9 Maverick Doctor are Reversing Alzheimer's, Dementia and Memory Loss

By Peggy Sarlin

Published by Online Publishing & Marketing, LLC

IMPORTANT CAUTION:

ISBN 978-1-4675-2369-1

Printed in the United States of America

ABOUT THE AUTHOR

Peggy Sarlin developed a special fascination with health and nutrition as a concerned mother of two who wanted to safeguard her family's well-being. She has written numerous articles on health and wellness for *Woman's World* magazine, a definitive book on an Asian superfood, and many successful pieces for Rodale and other leading health publishers. Most recently she penned the Special Report *The Secret Poison in Your Mouth*, warning of the deadly dangers of mercury amalgam dental fillings and root canals. When she's not writing about health, Sarlin is a scriptwriter for some of the best children's television shows on Disney, Nickelodeon and PBS and advises a national science competition for kids.

Contents

INTRODUCTION

If you or someone you love is struggling with Alzheimer's, I want to make you a promise. I guarantee that you'll be genuinely excited by the information you're about to discover.

Alzheimer's is such a tragic disease, and conventional medicine can only offer a few standard prescription drugs. Sadly, these medications are widely acknowledged to be almost useless, despite their dangerous side effects. Every day, thousands of people are told they have Alzheimer's and to go home and get their affairs in order. The overwhelming majority of doctors consider their situation hopeless.

But, in the words of Dr. Fred Pescatore, one of the many brilliant and innovative doctors I interviewed, "Don't resign yourself to your fate! There are so many things you can do!" This report is the story of the "many things" you can do, and the amazing possibilities for healing they can unleash.

Alzheimer's Patients Come Back to Life "Like A Watered Plant"

As I spoke to doctors, researchers, and caregivers around the country, I heard inspiring stories of patients deep into the decay of Alzheimer's "coming to life like a watered plant," "lighting up," and "becoming their old self again."

I listened to startling stories of people *nine years* into an Alzheimer's diagnosis, confounding their doctors with their high function. They were living independently, enjoying time with their families, and, sometimes, even driving. According to most doctors, by the ruthless arithmetic of Alzheimer's, they should either be dead by now or reduced to a pathetic shell.

What each success story had in common was someone who was determined to not give up: a husband, a wife, a son or daughter, or the patient him or herself. And their stubborn persistence drove to them to seek solutions outside the limited realm of conventional medicine.

Simple Steps that Produce Miracles in the Brain

From ancient natural remedies to groundbreaking new protocols, they found treatments that powerfully reversed the damage of Alzheimer's and woke up the brain's memory, clarity, and cognition.

Sometimes, the answer was as easy as a single supplement that you can buy in the grocery or pharmacy. Sometimes, the miracle came from a combination of simple steps taken under the care of a doctor trained in alternative medicine, whether naturopathy, integrative or functional medicine.

In almost every case, the process of reversing Alzheimer's required some trial and error, a bit of patience, and a lot of love. But when the right solution was found, the results could be dramatic and astonishingly fast.

You'll hear stories of patients recovering in weeks or even *days*, and getting right back to doing the *New York Times* crossword puzzle, running their businesses, and volunteering for their favorite charities.

Most importantly of all, their zest for life returned. They smiled, laughed, and joked around. They reclaimed their emotional stability. And, with a deeper appreciation than ever before, they relished spending time with family and friends.

Reversing the Brain's Aging Process with Targeted Supplements

As you read through these chapters, you'll keep seeing variations of this sentence: "*As you get older, your body's ability to <fill in the blank> declines.*" Aging is a complex process, and a lot of different things can go wrong. Any one of them – or all of them – can contribute to the onset of Alzheimer's.

That's why I've gathered a wealth of innovative ways to push back against the aging process in the brain. For instance, your brain's declining skill at managing **calcium** can be rekindled with the help of a new protein supplement called Prevagen.

Your brain's decreased capacity to metabolize **glucose**, its primary fuel, can be compensated for with ketones, which you'll get from coconut oil.

Your brain's dwindling supply of **Nerve Growth Factor**, which keeps brain neurons alive, can be sneakily re-stimulated by Lion's Mane, a gently effective medicinal mushroom.

And so on.

Secrets of the Most Brilliant, Natural-Minded Doctors

You won't find this information anywhere else. I've sought out the most accomplished, forward-thinking physicians around the country and pumped them for all their secrets about treating Alzheimer's.

And then I've shared their secrets with you.

You'll discover exactly how these dedicated doctors diagnose Alzheimer's. You'll hear their top priorities for treatment. And best of all, you'll receive priceless insider information: **the specific supplement regimen that these pioneering physicians advise their patients to follow**.

I think you'll be amazed at how many of these remedies have flown "beneath the radar," despite reams of studies that document their safety and effectiveness.

Fresh, New, Practical Information You Won't Find Anywhere Else

My quest is to bring you the most comprehensive, state-of-the-art information on reversing Alzheimer's. So I've also interviewed talented researchers who are working hard to develop the next wave of Alzheimer's treatments.

I've spoken to caregivers, who monitor the effects of remedies on their loved ones' behavior. Through their devoted care, they can see subtle changes, day by day, or even hour by hour.

And, of course, I've talked with Alzheimer's patients. I wanted to learn what it feels like to experience a reawakening brain, thanks to successful treatment.

Every person is different. You may respond to the remedies of a homeopathic doctor like Dr. Eric Udell. Someone else may find a breakthrough in the protocol of integrative physician Dr. Ronald Hoffman, or the hard-won wisdom of caregiver Joan Snow.

But the important thing is to stay optimistic and keep trying!

Reverse Parkinson's and Clear Up Brain Fog

Alzheimer's is a degenerative disease of the brain, and as I dug deeper into the research, I discovered that many Alzheimer's treatments also apply to Parkinson's, another brain disease. *If you know someone with Parkinson's, please tell them about the information here.* They urgently need to discover these healing tools, which have the potential to transform their quality of life.

You don't need an Alzheimer's diagnosis to benefit from these powerful brain-boosters. If you're worried about fading memory and decreased mental function, these supplements will work for you, too. You can take them in lower doses to help prevent Alzheimer's, and to chase away brain fog and memory loss.

Anyone who's lived with Alzheimer's knows that it can be an unbearable nightmare of loss. As you begin your journey away from Alzheimer's and towards renewed hope, take courage from the wise old saying: *"The heart that truly loves never forgets."*

And now, let me introduce you to the people who graciously gave me their time for interviews. I owe them all my profound gratitude.

My Heartfelt Thanks To...

Dr. Fred Pescatore, M.D.: President of the International and American Association of Clinical Nutritionists; former Associate Medical Director of The Atkins Center for Complementary Medicine; founder, Partners in Integrative medicine (NYC); author of five health and nutrition books, including the *New York Times* bestseller, *The Hamptons Diet*.

Dr. Jacob Teitelbaum, M.D.: director of The Annapolis Center for Effective CFS/Fibromyalgia Therapies. He battled chronic fatigue Syndrome and fibromyalgia while attending medical school in the mid-70's. In his struggle to heal, he discovered treatments that were unknown to the medical community and began a quest that became his life's passion -- helping those who suffer from these debilitating illnesses. The treatment program he developed has helped tens of thousands of sufferers reclaim the vitality CFS/FMS once robbed from their lives.

Dr. Farhang Khosh, N.D.: received his Doctorate of Naturopathic Medicine from Bastyr University, a nationally accredited naturopathic medical school in Seattle. Dr. Khosh practices with Natural Medical Care in Lawrence, Kansas.

Dr. Ronald Hoffman, M.D.: recognized as one of America's foremost complementary medicine practitioners. He is founder and Medical Director of the Hoffman Center in New York City, author of numerous books and articles for the public and for health professionals, and is host of the popular nationally-syndicated radio program "Health Talk". He is active in several medical professional organizations, and is a past President of the country's largest organization of complementary and alternative doctors, the American College for Advancement in Medicine (ACAM).

Dr. Marty Hinz, M.D.: medical doctor; founder, NeuroResearch Clinic

Dr. Tara Peyman, N.D.: licensed naturopathic doctor in the state of Arizona. Dr. Peyman's primary passion is the homeopathic and integrative treatment of bipolar disorder and mental illness. She practices with Arizona Natural Health Center in Tempe, Arizona.

Dr. Eric Udell, N.D.: Dr. Udell has a strong reputation for excellence in homeopathy and for his ability to tackle challenging cases. He is an Assistant Professor of Homeopathy at Southwest College of Naturopathic Medicine and practices in Arizona.

Dr. Gary Klingsberg, DO, M.D.: specializes in family practice, preventive medicine and occupational medicine in Englewood, New Jersey.

Mark Underwood: biological researcher, founder of Quincy Bioscience, maker of Prevagen

Dr. Gail Lowenstein, M.D.: board-certified in Internal Medicine, Geriatrics, Hospice and Palliative Medicine, Holistic Medicine, and has added qualifications in Functional Medicine. She currently practices in New York State.

Dr. Jeffrey Morrison, M.D., C.N.S.: Director of the Morrison Medical Center in New York City. Dr. Jeffrey Morrison is a medical doctor who champions a nutritional approach to healthcare as well as preventing and reversing degenerative diseases. Dr. Morrison's specific treatments are aimed at enhancing the body's ability to heal and detoxify itself. These safe, non-toxic and non-invasive therapies are proving to be more powerful than conventional treatments, which utilize often dangerous drugs and surgeries.

Thomas J. Wilson, Pharm.D.: Founder of Cape Apothecary in Annapolis, Maryland, Dr. Wilson specializes in Compounding, Hormone Replacement Therapy, Herbal and Homeopathic Medicine, Nutritional Supplements, as well as Veterinary Products. Cape Apothecary has been serving the local community for over 35 years.

Joan Snow: caregiver to her father, a longtime Alzheimer's patient

Coleen Melsted: daughter of Alzheimer's patient

Carolyn: Alzheimer's patient

I also owe a special debt of thanks for his help to **Dr. Vincent Fortanasce**.

Dr. Vincent Fortanasce: Board-certified in neurology and rehabilitation, psychiatrist and renowned bioethicist, Dr. Vincent Fortanasce is a clinical professor of neurology at the University of Southern California. Named one of the best physicians in America, he is the author of *The Anti-Alzheimer's Prescription*.

Chapter 1

16 Facts About Alzheimer's

Before we delve into how to reverse Alzheimer's, let's establish some basic facts.

Fact One: Alzheimer's is the most common form of dementia. Approximately 5.1 million Americans and 24 million people worldwide now have Alzheimer's. As the Baby Boomers generation ages, experts fear that Alzheimer's will become a public health catastrophe.

Fact Two: Alzheimer's is not the only cause of dementia. Vascular dementia, which is caused by blocked arteries to the brain, is the second most common type. Other forms include dementia with Lewy bodies, fronto-temporal dementia, and dementia brought on by a stroke.

Fact Three: Alzheimer's disease is named after Dr. Alois Alzheimer. In 1906, Dr. Alzheimer discovered changes in the brain tissue of a woman who had died at age 55 of an unusual mental illness. Her symptoms included memory loss, language problems, and strange behavior.

Fact Four: Dr. Alzheimer examined her brain and found two abnormalities, which we now understand are characteristic of Alzheimer's: **plaques and tangles**. Parts of the brain were covered with sticky plaque made of **beta-amyloid protein**. And **neurofibrillary tangles**, which are messy bundles of degenerating nerve endings, also appeared throughout the brain.

Fact Five: As the amyloid plaques and neurofibrillary tangles grow, nerve cells in the brain (**neurons**) lose their ability to communicate and begin to die.

Fact Six: Alzheimer's usually develops in people over 65. But about 5 percent of patients contract early-onset Alzheimer's, which can strike as early as age 30. Early-onset Alzheimer's often runs in families, and is linked to changes in one of three known genes inherited from a parent.

Fact Seven: The risk of developing late-onset Alzheimer's is increased by one genetic risk factor: the **apolipoprotein E (APOE) gene** found on chromosome 19. But even if you carry that genetic factor, you won't necessarily develop the disease.

Fact Eight: Alzheimer's progresses in stages.

• In **stage 1**, which is mild Alzheimer's, patients exhibit memory loss, language problems, personality changes, lack of focus, and diminished judgment. Stage 1 lasts one to two years.

- In **stage 2**, or moderate Alzheimer's, patients are disoriented, have serious memory problems, insomnia, aggression, agitation and wandering at sundown, and may need help with tasks of daily life. Stage 2 also lasts one to two years.

- In **stage 3,** or severe Alzheimer's, patients can no longer recognize people, have difficulty speaking, and are eventually bedridden. This stage can last about six years. The average patient lives about 8.2 years after being diagnosed.

Fact Nine: We don't yet understand the exact cause of Alzheimer's, but it appears to be a mix of genetic, environmental, and lifestyle factors. Obesity, hypertension and abnormal blood lipids are known to increase the risk.

Fact Ten: Alzheimer's strikes in the hippocampus, which is vital for memory and mood. As plaques and tangles accumulate in the hippocampus, its ability to store and retrieve memory declines.

Fact Eleven: Alzheimer's is strongly associated with oxidative stress, or "brain rust." Typically, Alzheimer's brains have weak antioxidant protection against attack from free radicals.

Fact Twelve: Alzheimer's is strongly linked to inflammation, or "brain on fire." High inflammatory markers can be good predictors of developing Alzheimer's.

Fact Thirteen: Alzheimer's is associated with high levels of homocysteine in the blood. Homocysteine is an amino acid produced by the body, which can damage the hippocampus and increase inflammation, if it's present in excess amounts.

Fact Fourteen: The medical establishment agrees that prescription drugs for Alzheimer's can only help modestly, at best. Here's how the U.S. government's National Institute of Aging describes them:

"Four medications are approved by the U.S. Food and Drug Administration to treat Alzheimer's. Donepezil (Aricept®), rivastigmine (Exelon®), and galantamine (Razadyne®) are used to treat mild to moderate Alzheimer's (donepezil can be used for severe Alzheimer's as well). Memantine (Namenda®) is used to treat moderate to severe Alzheimer's. These drugs work by regulating neurotransmitters (the chemicals that transmit messages between neurons). They may help maintain thinking, memory, and speaking skills, and help with certain behavioral problems. **However, these drugs don't change the underlying disease process, are effective for some but not all people, and may help only for a limited time**."

Fact Fifteen: Most Alzheimer's medications can have dangerous side effects. Ironically, these side effects can mimic the symptoms of Alzheimer's, such as depression, mood changes, confusion and hallucinations.

Fact Sixteen: Alzheimer's *can* be reversed. You don't have to resign yourself to suffering, or to watching someone you love with all your heart and soul fade away. If you enlarge your scope beyond the standard prescription drugs, you may very well be stunned by how successfully you can restore memory, focus, clarity and zest for life.

To get started, all you have to do is turn the page.

Sources:

National Institute on Aging
Alzheimer's Disease Education and Referral Center
www.nia.nih.gov/alzheimers

The Better Brain Book
David Perlmutter, M.D., FACN and Carol Colman
Riverhead Books, 2004

The Anti-Alzheimer's Prescription
Vincent Fortanasce, M.D.
Gotham Books, 2008

The Alzheimer's Prevention Plan
Patrick Holford with Shane Heaton and Deborah Colson
Piatkus Books, 2005

Chapter 2

The Coconut Oil Miracle:
How Dr. Mary Newport Reversed Her Husband's Alzheimer's in 37 Days

If you need inspiration about reversing Alzheimer's, you'll be delighted by the story of Dr. Mary Newport and her husband Steve. It's a love story, of course, starring a devoted wife who refused to let her husband fade away without a fight. It's got a great cast, an exciting plot, and best of all, it's got a happy ending!

Our story begins as Steve Newport, an accountant who managed his wife's successful medical practice, started to feel his mind slipping away. He forgot appointments, misplaced his wallet, and got lost driving home. And, for the first time ever, he made mistakes with the payroll and missed a tax deadline. Steve's razor-sharp mind was melting away...and he was only 52 years old!

Sadly, by age 58, Steve had deteriorated so badly, he could no longer function. His neurologist put him on Aricept, Namenda and Exelon, but nothing seemed to help. The dynamic man who loved to cook for his daughters and go kayaking in the wilderness had disappeared. In his place was a lost soul, who wandered aimlessly around the house in one shoe, and, sometimes, didn't even recognize his family.

Mary was heartbroken. Pouring out her pain in her journal, she wrote, "It has been a nightmare to watch his decline. Every night, we hold each other before we go to sleep and I wonder how many more times we will get to do this."

"I didn't know what was happening to me. I was confused," Steve said, looking back at this tragic time.

In August, 2007, Steve stopped eating and suddenly lost ten pounds, Mary knew she had to take drastic action. But what could she do? She tried to enroll Steve in clinical trials of experimental drugs, but nobody wanted to take him. Steve's condition was too severe.

In fact, Steve was so far gone that he couldn't remember the season, month or day of the week. On the Mini Mental Status Exam (MMSR), he scored only 14 out of 30, a sign of severe dementia. To make matters worse, his MRI indicated that his hippocampus had withered away.

His brain's frontal and parietal lobes also showed damage. And, as if to seal his fate, Steve tested positive for the genetic marker of early onset Alzheimer's.

Just A Spoonful of Miracles Makes the Alzheimer's Go Away

In May 2008, Mary worked deep into the night, researching experimental drugs. She discovered something that startled her with hope. Half the patients on a new drug showed memory improvement!

"Most drugs talk about slowing the progression of the disease, but you never hear the word 'improvement.' Right then I knew I had to find out more," Mary explained to the St. Petersburg Times.

As Mary delved into the research, she learned that the drug's main ingredient was MCT oil, which derives from coconuts.

Sometimes despair can drive inspiration. With nothing left to lose, Mary drove to the health food store and bought a jar of non-hydrogenated, extra virgin coconut oil.

The next morning, she secretly added two teaspoons of coconut oil to Steve's oatmeal. And then, she prayed. "I prayed harder than I'd ever prayed in my life," she said.

After breakfast, Mary drove Steve to his medical appointment, where he took the same Mini Mental Status Exam that he'd taken the day before. The results were stunning. Steve *scored 28% higher* than he had on yesterday's test!

"It was like the oil kicked in and he could think clearly again," Mary told the St. Petersburg Times. "We were ecstatic."

Mary's prayers were answered. Every morning, she gave Steve coconut oil, and every day he showed remarkable improvement. By the fifth day, his natural good humor had returned and he could feel "the fog lift."

You can see for yourself Steve's amazing progress by looking at three pictures he drew. The day before Steve started taking coconut oil, he drew a picture of a clock that was so pathetic, it brought tears to his wife's eyes. Two weeks after he began taking coconut oil, Steve drew another clock. Look at the difference. And on Day 37 of his coconut oil routine, Steve drew the third clock you see here. The miracle had happened! The light bulb in Steve's brain had been switched on.

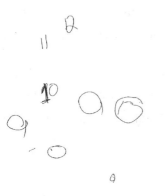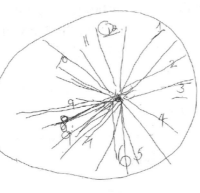

Clock #1 - The day before starting coconut oil.

Clock #2 - Two weeks after starting coconut oil.

Clock #3 - Thirty-seven days after starting coconut oil.

Today, Steve Newport Enjoys a Full Life

On May 21, 2011, Dr. Mary Newport wrote a grateful entry on her website, titled "Steve's 3rd Anniversary." "Today is the 3rd Anniversary of the day, May 21, 2008, when he began to take coconut oil and saw the improvements that changed both of our lives," she wrote.

And what a change it's been! Today, Steve has so much energy, he jogs every day. He volunteers at the local hospital, and takes care of chores around the house, including mowing the lawn. His mood is cheerful, and he likes to crack jokes. His tremor has vanished. His mind is so focused that he enjoys reading articles in *Scientific American*, and telling Mary the details of what he learned. And, of course, he loves to spend time with his family, including his precious grandson.

What's the magic formula that switched on Steve's mind? If it sounds simple, that's because it *is* simple. Every day, Steve takes a mixture of MCT oil and coconut oil. His dosage is three tablespoons, three times a day. He also takes a fourth dose at bedtime of two tablespoons, which was added when he was having some difficulty sleeping.

What Makes Coconut Oil Work

To understand the science behind Steve's miracle, let's take a look at what fuels your brain. You may be surprised to learn that the brain is the most metabolically active organ in the body. It accounts for two percent of your body's mass, but for 20 per cent of its basal metabolic rate. To power up all that activity, your brain needs lots of fuel. And when you're healthy, that fuel comes from glucose, a blood sugar.

But brains that are afflicted with Alzheimer's have trouble metabolizing glucose. And without a constant resupply of glucose, brain neurons start to die.

Fortunately, under the right conditions, your body is capable of creating a back-up source of high-energy brain fuel. That fuel is *ketones*, a type of fat that your liver can extract from MCT oil and coconut oil.

Do you recognize the term ketones? You probably know it from the famous Atkins Diet. The Atkins' low-carb, high-fat eating plan forces the body into a natural state of *ketosis*, in which elevated levels of ketone bodies are released into the bloodstream. In this state, the body burns fat, instead of carbohydrates, so you lose weight.

Scientists have been studying the effects of ketones on the brain for years. In fact, Dr. Newport's website links to twenty scientific papers documenting the positive effect of ketones on mental function. One important study found that a ketone-inducing diet produced a *39% increase* in blood flow! Another study revealed that a brain fueled by ketones produces 25% more energy than a glucose-fueled brain.

I spoke to Dr. Eric Udell, a naturopathic doctor in Arizona, about ketones and Alzheimer's. Dr. Udell advises his Alzheimer's patients to take MCT oil, which is derived from coconut oil. (MCT stands for medium chain triglycerides.)

"Glucose is the main source of brain energy," Dr. Udell explained to me. "Brain cells are not as adaptable as other parts of the body. When they become less efficient at using glucose for energy, MCT provides an alternative fuel that allows them to function better."

"I would make MCT oil a standard component of an Alzheimer's supplement regimen. It's safe and non-toxic," Dr. Udell told me. A medical grade MCT is available by prescription, he noted.

Dr. Jeffrey Morrison of the Morrison Center in New York echoes Dr. Udell's views on the importance of ketones for Alzheimer's patients. "Anybody with Alzheimer's should use coconut oil," he told me. "It's super-important to get MCTs – the medium-chain triglycerides in coconut oil – two or three times a day."

And, of course, Dr. Mary Newport is convinced of the healing power of ketones on Alzheimer's-damaged brains. She sees the evidence every day, when she looks at Steve.

Why Dr. Mary Newport is a Hero to Families Everywhere

Dr. Newport is a busy woman, with lots of responsibilities. She's a pediatrician with a specialty in the care of sick and premature newborns. Currently, she is the director of the Neonatal Intensive Care Unit at Spring Hill Regional Hospital in Florida. Previously, she served as medical director at Mease Hospital Dunedin, where she founded a Neonatal Intensive Care Unit in 1987.

But despite her whirlwind life, Dr. Newport always finds another hour in her day to spread the word about coconut oil. She started a website, *coconutketones.com*, where she shares her advice and the latest research. Dr. Newport's goal is to let families know about coconut oil, and to spur further research into its potential. As of February, 2011, her website had gotten 700,000 hits!

She's written a book, **Alzheimer's Disease: What If There Were a Cure?,** telling her husband's story and examining the research on ketones. And she regularly speaks to medical groups, newspapers and television shows about the healing power of coconut oil.

Who knows how many lives she has changed? The story of Mary and Steve Newport has become a legend in Alzheimer's chat rooms, and an inspiration to families everywhere struggling with the ravages of this cruel disease. Dr. Newport's loving determination to not give up, and to keep looking for a better solution can bring hope and motivation to anyone touched by Alzheimer's.

"I think (Dr. Newport) is quite courageous. Most people give up when they are facing severe Alzheimer's, but she feels she's got significant improvement," said Dr. Richard Veech, who's been studying ketones for more than 40 years. Dr. Veech is chief of the lab of metabolic control at the National Institutes of Health, and helps to advise Mary in her personal study of ketones.

"I've got living proof that this will help people," Dr. Newport said. "I want to just tell everybody about this. It may help them improve, too."

And word is getting out. Here's the heartwarming story of a husband and wife in Australia whose lives were in crisis until they discovered coconut oil through Dr. Newport.

How Cassie Got Her Husband Back

Ian Blair Hamilton, 64, was used to long, challenging days as the managing director of a health product company. But lately, he found his mind wobbling. His father had Alzheimer's, and he was horrified to recognize the signs in himself. Forgetting words. Getting confused about what to do next. Depression.

At first, he tried to deny it was happening. But as his condition worsened, he confided in his wife, Cassie. "I was so scared I'd be left with someone I had to take care of," said Cassie, in a video the couple filmed for YouTube.

Cassie plunged into researching Alzheimer's on the Internet. When she discovered Dr. Mary Newport's site, she knew she had to try giving coconut oil to Ian.

The results were dramatic - and amazingly fast. Within a week, Ian's depression had lifted.

Ian's mind is now as "sharp as ever," he says, and his creative ability is operating full blast.

"I got my husband back," says Cassie.

Every day, Ian takes two tablespoons of coconut oil with kefir and blueberries, like a smoothie. And he and Cassie use coconut oil for their cooking.

Ian's story highlights the importance of treating Alzheimer's as soon as possible. Once extensive physical damage is done to the brain, complete recovery is much more difficult. But if you take fast action at the disease's onset, you could very well stop it cold, before any permanent injury occurs.

Ian feels grateful that he discovered coconut oil within months of his first symptoms. "We nipped it at the right moment. I got back to normal," says Ian.

Dr. Newport's Advice on Using Coconut Oil

On Dr. Newport's website, **coconutketones.com**, she offers lots of practical advice on how to use coconut oil in your daily routine.

Here are some important tips to help you get started.

- Buy coconut oil that is non-hydrogenated with no transfat. Products labeled "virgin," "organic," or "unrefined," tend to be more expensive, and give off the odor of coconut. The less expensive products, which are called "refined," or "all natural" or "RBD" have no odor.

- The least expensive brand that Dr. Newport has found is LouAna, which sells at Walmart for about $5.44 per quart.

- You may also want to use MCT oil. MCT stands for medium chain triglycerides, which are part of the coconut oil. You can buy MCT oil at health food stores or online. MCT oil does not store in the body as fat. Instead, it's quickly converted to energy, and may be helpful for losing weight. A medical-grade MCT oil is available by prescription.

- Coconut oil contains 117 – 120 calories per tablespoon, which is about the same as other oils. Keep its caloric content in mind, if weight is an issue.

- Coconut oil contains **omega-6 fatty acids**. Your body also needs **omega-3 fatty acids**. You can get your omega-3 supply by eating salmon twice a week, or taking fish oil or flax oil capsules, 2-3 per day. Walnuts and walnut oil also contain omega-3 fatty acids.

- Coconut milk, flaked or grated coconut, and fresh coconut are all good sources of coconut oil.

- If you overwhelm your digestive system by taking too much oil too fast, you could experience indigestion, cramps, or diarrhea. Start with 1 teaspoon of coconut oil or MCT oil per meal. Slowly work up your level to 4-6 tablespoons a day, spread out over 2–4 meals.

- If you mix MCT oil and coconut oil, you'll get a higher and steadier supply of ketones. Dr. Newport's suggested formula is to mix 16 ounces of MCT oil plus 12 ounces of coconut oil in a quart jar. You can keep the jar at room temperature, where it will stay liquid.

- Get creative with your use of coconut oil. Add it to oatmeal and hot cereals. Use it instead of butter on your bread, vegetables and pasta. Stir it into your soups and sauces. Add it to smoothies, yogurt or kefir. Add coconut oil to your salad dressings. Stir fry or sauté with coconut, adding peanut oil over medium heat. Add flaked or grated coconut to cereal, salads, and yogurt.

A Model Confesses the Secret of Her Beautiful Skin and Hair

And don't be surprised if you notice some other terrific benefits from your daily dose of coconut oil. I was fascinated to discover an interview with famed Victoria's Secret model, Miranda Kerr. She claimed that the secret of her glowing skin and glossy hair is coconut oil!

The 28-year-old beauty said, "I will not go a day without coconut oil. I personally take four tablespoons per day, either on my salads, in my cooking or in my cups of green tea." After Miranda Kerr confessed her beauty secret, sales of coconut oil skyrocketed by 50%, according to a British newspaper.

Miranda Kerr's outer glow may derive from an inner glow of robust good health. Along with beautiful skin and hair, non-hydrogenated coconut oil provides an amazing array of other advantages:

- May improve your cholesterol readings, raising your HDL ("good") cholesterol and lowering your LDL ("bad") levels.

- Contains lauric acid, which has antimicrobial properties. Lauric acid may inhibit growth of certain bacteria, fungus, yeast, viruses and protozoa.

- Improves insulin secretion and utilization of blood glucose.

- Assists digestion and absorption of other nutrients including vitamins, minerals, and amino acids.

- Reduces inflammation and helps protect against osteoporosis.

- Helps protect the body from breast, colon, and other cancers.

Can Parkinson's Disease Be Reversed With Coconut Oil?

Like Alzheimer's, Parkinson's is a neurodegenerative disease. And evidence suggests that Parkinson's patients may also get a big boost by raising their ketones levels.

Dr. Theodore VanItallie of Columbia University conducted a promising small study in 2005 with five Parkinson's patients. He put them on a ketogenic diet for a month. Every participant enjoyed improved ability to walk, and reduced tremors and stiffness, on average, by as much as 43%.

"Our study was very successful for our patients," said Dr. VanItallie, who hopes that larger-scale studies will continue his research.

In fact, Dr. Richard Veech is now conducting a Parkinson's study in Oxford, England at John Radcliffe Hospital. Dr. Veech's study will examine ketones' effect on twenty Parkinson's patients over the short term.

It's possible that someday ketones will prove to be the key to healing any illness in which the body can't process glucose. Type I and II diabetes, multiple sclerosis, Huntington's disease and Lou Gehrig's disease may all eventually be treated with ketones.

A big believer in the power of ketones is Hollywood producer Jim Abrahams, who's famous for his *Airplane* movies. He started the Charlie Foundation to promote the ketogenic diet, after it cured his infant son of the nightmare of constant epileptic seizures.

Axona, A Medical Milkshake for the Brain

And now there's Axona, a vanilla milkshake that's classified as a medical food for Alzheimer's. Axona is available through prescription, although not all doctors are willing to prescribe it.

Axona contains a medium-chain triglyceride (MCT) called caprylic triglyceride, which is derived from coconut oil. Here's how Accera Inc., the Colorado-based manufacturer of Axona, explains its effect:

Axona® is a prescription medical food intended for the clinical dietary management of the metabolic processes associated with mild to moderate Alzheimer's disease. Axona addresses the decline in glucose metabolism—a well-characterized feature of Alzheimer's disease. Taking Axona produces ketone bodies—which the brain can use as an energy source—to manage glucose hypometabolism. Patients with mild to moderate Alzheimer's disease taking Axona demonstrated improved cognitive function as measured by ADAS-Cog.

Axona comes in a 217-calorie packet that can be mixed with any type of liquid in a shaker cup or blender. As a medical food, Axona doesn't require FDA approval. The price is $70 to $90 for a one-month supply. Insurance usually doesn't cover the cost.

Axona has sparked a hot debate in the medical community about its value. *The Wall Street Journal* and *ABC News* both ran recent articles about Axona, in which some researchers praised its novel approach. Others blasted Axona as "snake oil."

"It's an expense to your budget with limited evidence that it will do any good," said William Thies, Chief Medical and Scientific Officer for the Alzheimer's Association.

"This is just expensive coconut oil," said Dr. Roger Brumback, professor of neurology at the Creighton University School of Medicine.

Glenn Smith, PhD., writing at the Mayo Clinic's website, answered a reader's question about Axona by noting, "It's not clear what benefit, if any, Axona provides." Dr. Smith stated that the Alzheimer's Association "disputes the notion that Alzheimer's disease causes nutritional deficiencies and requires a medical food... Until more is known, the Alzheimer's Association doesn't recommend the use of medical foods, including Axona, for the treatment of Alzheimer's disease."

But don't give that gloomy report to Chris Freeman and his 89-year-old mother, Peg Kinnison.

Axona Brought His Mother's Memory Back

Peg Kinnison spent forty years teaching in Michigan and Washington, D.C., enjoying the give and take of being around people.

But when Alzheimer's struck her in her eighties, she withdrew into herself. Her doctor prescribed two of the most common Alzheimer's drugs, Aricept and Namenda.

Chris Freeman, her devoted son, wasn't satisfied with the results. A former biochemist, Chris plowed into researching additional supplements for his mother.

Chris's investigation led him to Axona. But when he asked his mother's geriatrician to prescribe it, the doctor refused.

Chris persisted, and convinced Kinnison's internist to write a prescription. Axona's positive effect on his mother's behavior was immediate, says Chris.

In fact, Chris told the *Cleveland Plain Dealer* that Axona has been a miracle. "Her memory has come back, she eats more, she's willing to do more." And, she's become "more lively and talkative again."

Peg Kinnison said she noticed the improvement in herself, too. She finds herself taking part in conversations again, instead of being a silent observer.

Chris Freeman told the *Plain Dealer* that he "believes it's important to be a strong advocate for a loved one's health care and to stay open-minded about possible treatments."

He's determined to stay on top of the latest developments in Alzheimer's treatment and to make sure his mother gets the best care.

His grateful mother says Chris's devotion inspires her. "Here's someone who's really trying to help me, so I have to try."

Your Best Choice: Coconut Oil, MCT Oil, or Axona?

Coconut oil, MCT oil and Axona all contain the same compound: Medium-Chain Triglycerides. Your liver can convert MCTs into ketone bodies, which provide a high-energy, alternate fuel for your brain.

It's important to realize that MCTs come in different types. Axona contains caprylidene, which can't be found in either coconut oil or MCT oil. MCT oil contains a much higher percentage of caprylic acid and capric acid than does coconut oil. And coconut oil is 48% composed of lauric acid, which is found in neither Axona nor MCT oil.

The bottom line: each of these supplements contains different MCTs that may be helpful. Your body may respond better to one supplement over the other. Or you may feel best by using two of them, or even all three.

Cost will probably be a factor for you. An online site called Alzheimer's Weekly (alzheimersweekly.com), ran a cost analysis of these three supplements. They concluded that in order to get 20 grams of MCTs from Axona, you'll need to spend $3.00 a day. 20 grams of MCTs from MCT oil costs 84 cents a day. And 20 grams of MCTs from coconut oil costs 22 cents a day.

Axona conducted its study on patients who were given one 20 gram MCT dose a day. But Alzheimer's patients may need to get an MCT boost throughout the day. Otherwise, their ketones levels may drop too low.

So should you take Axona in the morning, and then take coconut oil and/or MCT oil with your later meals? Dr. Mary Newport wrote a comment on Alzheimer's Weekly's website, explaining her thoughts on keeping ketones levels steady.

"After studying Steve's ketone levels with both coconut oil and MCT oil, I began mixing MCT and coconut oil together to try to get higher peak levels from the MCT oil and also longer duration of ketone levels from the coconut oil, so that he would have ketones circulating 24/7.

Axona can only recommend taking one 20 gram MCT dose a day because that is what they studied. The ketones levels from one dose peak between 60 and 90 minutes and are virtually gone within 3 hours. Hopefully, they will continue their studies and look at two and three doses a day."

Ketones offer genuine hope for Alzheimer's sufferers. You can experiment and see what options work best for you. Who knows what exciting healing possibilities you'll find? Renewed mental vigor may be waiting inside the coconut oil you mix into your oatmeal, or the MCT oil you mix into your tea.

As Dr. Mary Newport says, "All I'm asking is to investigate this further. After living through Alzheimer's, anything that can stabilize or help improve (your loved one) will be worth every drop."

Sources:

Dr. Mary Newport's website:
http://coconutketones.com/

Dr. Mary Newport's blog:
http://coconutketones.blogspot.com/

Alzheimer's Disease: What If There Was a Cure?
The Story of Ketones
by Mary T. Newport, MD
From Basic Health Publications, Inc.
Available on Amazon

Sources on coconut oil:

Tampa Bay Times
"Doctor says an oil lessened Alzheimer's effects on her husband"
By Eve Hosley-Moore, Times Correspondent
Wednesday, October 29, 2008
http://www.tampabay.com/news/aging/article879333.ece

Daily Mail, United Kingdom
"Victoria's Secret? Coconut oil... Sales boom as model Miranda Kerr reveals daily dose of 'healthy fat' is key to her beauty"
By Tamara Cohen
25th August 2011

www.dailymail.co.uk/femail/article-2029573/Victorias-Secret-supermodel-Miranda-Kerrs-coconut-oil-beauty-secret.html#ixzz1hyCknZ6T

Alzheimer's Weekly
The Keto-Dementia Diet
http://alzheimersweekly.com/content/keto-dementia-diet

Coconut Research Center
www.coconutresearchcenter.org

On Axona:
http://about-axona.com/

ABC News
"Doctors Debate Effectiveness of Alzheimer's Milkshake"
Carrie Gann
August 31, 2011
http://abcnews.go.com/Health/alzheimers-milkshake-treatment-snake-oil/story?id=14421476#.Tvz88Ep4Ufo

Mayo Clinic
"Axona: Medical food to treat Alzheimer's"
www.mayoclinic.com/health/axona/an01992

Cleveland Plain Dealer
"Axona, a 'medical food,' is tried by an Alzheimer's patient: Healthy Cleveland"
By Brie Zeltner

Tuesday, August 11, 2009
http://www.cleveland.com/healthfit/index.ssf/2009/08/axona_a_medical_food_is_tried.html

The Wall Street Journal
"Fueling the Brain with a Milkshake"
Laura Johannes
August 30, 2011
online.wsj.com/article/SB10001424053111904199404576538582281006022.html

Alzheimer's Weekly

"New Clinical Trial Results for Axona"

http://alzheimersweekly.com/content/new-clinical-trial-results-axona

Axona, MCT and Coconut Oil: Differences and Benefits

http://alzheimersweekly.com/content/axona-mct-coconut-oil-differences-benefits

http://www.alzheimersweekly.com/content/axona-mct-coconut-oil-differences-benefits#comment

Interviews with Dr. Eric Udell and Dr. Jeffrey Morrison

Chapter 3

Can A Jellyfish's Glow Light Up Your Brain?

When Mark Underwood was a college undergraduate, he read an article about an unlucky swimmer that fired up his imagination. The swimmer had gotten stung by jellyfish, and then developed symptoms like those seen in multiple sclerosis.

As a neurochemistry student, Mark tried to puzzle out what had happened. If the jellyfish can provoke multiple sclerosis symptoms, how does it protect itself from the disease?

The problem was an interesting intellectual challenge. But Mark also had an emotional connection to it, too.

"My mother has multiple sclerosis," Mark told me, in a phone interview. "And my grandfather had Alzheimer's. So I was very interested in studying these issues."

Today, Mark Underwood is a neuroscience researcher and the co-founder of Quincy Bioscience. And he's more fascinated than ever by jellyfish and their impact on human health.

In fact, Quincy Bioscience makes a supplement for brain health called Prevagen. And its unique active ingredient is apoaequorin, which was first discovered in jellyfish.

A number of doctors I interviewed told me that they're recommending Prevagen to their Alzheimer's patients. They consider it a valuable new addition to their tool kit for patients with memory problems.

Prevagen's researchers say its benefits may be seen as early as the first week. But most people feel the improvement between 30 and 90 days after they start taking it.

The Unique Compound That Keeps Brain Cells Alive Longer

Prevagen may soon become much more popular. It recently went mass market, appearing on the shelves of Walgreens and Rite Aid. In fact, 14,000 nationwide locations now carry it, including many health food stores. And the number of outlets continues to grow every month.

What's fueling its success? According to pre-clinical research, apoaequorin is the only compound ever laboratory-proven to keep brain cells alive longer.

Researchers at the University of Wisconsin-Milwaukee studied apoaequorin's ability to protect brain cells, using a model of ischemic stroke (stroke that occurs when an artery to the brain is blocked). The researchers found up to a **50% reduction in cellular death**, when compared to non-apoaequorin treated cells.

An aging brain can lose 30,000 to 50,000 brain cells *a day*. Prevagen's protection may prove enormously important in safeguarding the brain health of aging Baby Boomers. And it offers real hope to Alzheimer's sufferers and their families.

Prevagen Promotes Clearer Thinking, Protects Memories

I asked Mark Underwood to explain how Prevagen works. People who use it often report better focus and memory, and improved mental clarity and word recall. And the benefits don't stop there. Some Prevagen users say they sleep better and feel greater energy, too.

So how does a jellyfish protein promote all that?

"As I studied jellyfish, I learned they contain a protein called apoaequorin. This protein is part of what makes them glow in the dark," Mark explained.

I told Mark that I already knew from my reading that apoaequorin was first isolated in 1962 by Dr. Osamu Shimomura. In 2008, he and two other researchers won the Nobel Prize in Chemistry for this discovery, which turned out to have many medical applications.

"That's right," said Mark. "Now what interested me was that this protein from jellyfish has the ability to bind calcium ions. You and I have calcium-binding proteins that we make naturally. They keep our brain cells working properly and communicating."

"But as we get older, especially after age 40, our ability to make these calcium-binding proteins slows down. And if we can't make enough, eventually this shortage will lead to brain cell death in Alzheimer's and Parkinson's patients. And in healthy people, too."

"In the mid-1980s, Alzheimer's researchers did autopsies on Alzheimer's patients. They looked at the brain and saw damage caused by calcium ions."

"So I put these two ideas together. The jellyfish contains a protein that binds calcium ions. And as people get older, they lose the ability to make calcium-binding proteins. Why not help people with jellyfish protein?"

"I wrote a long paper about it as an undergraduate. Then I shelved the idea for a while. In 2004, we started Quincy Bioscience, and now we make Prevagen."

I asked Mark about his emphasis on calcium. Many experts feel that Alzheimer's is caused by inflammation and/or the growth of a sticky plaque on the brain. Yet, Mark attributed Alzheimer's damage to calcium mismanagement in the brain. Wasn't that a completely different approach?

"Calcium modulates inflammation in the brain," Mark explained. "If you have too much unregulated calcium, you'll get too much inflammation."

"And if you look at the plaque associated with Alzheimer's, it drills little holes into neurons. Those holes allow calcium to enter the cells and leak in. And when calcium enters, it causes the brain cell to die."

"You can have the calcium problem with or without the plaque," he continued. "I don't think the plaques matter that much. A lot of other things in the brain can go wrong that cause calcium levels to rise. Head injuries, diet, stress, chemicals, toxins…Plaque could be one of ten things going on."

"It's like electricity in a computer. If it's turned off, the computer won't work. But if you have too much, it can cause the computer to short-circuit. If the brain has too much calcium, it short-circuits."

Do people lose their calcium balance at different rates, I asked.

"There's a full spectrum of how quickly people lose their calcium balance," Mark replied. "You can have a forgetful person who's fifty years old, but doesn't have Alzheimer's. And then, you can have people like athletes who had a head trauma that, over time, disrupted calcium balance. NFL players are 17 times more likely to get Alzheimer's, because of brain damage. Or you can be healthy as a horse at age forty, and feeling the effects of a car accident from when you were twenty."

Calcium Imbalance Provokes Alzheimer's, Parkinson's, Huntington's

"Now realize, calcium isn't bad. And calcium imbalance doesn't have anything to do with how much calcium you take in. The problem is your calcium is mismanaged."

"Autopsies of brains with schizophrenia, Huntington's, Parkinson's, and Alzheimer's, all show the need to maintain calcium balance."

"In Alzheimer's patients, the damage forms in the hippocampus first. In the Parkinson's patients, they lose the ability to make dopamine. You have the same calcium imbalance, but it's manifesting differently, because of where the damage manifests first."

"If people are presenting with memory loss, depression and tremors, there's only one thing that contributes to all three. That's a calcium imbalance in the brain."

"From a practical perspective, they have a problem that needs to be resolved, whether you call it Alzheimer's or Parkinson's. Fix the calcium, and all these symptoms start to resolve. And we can keep brain cells alive longer."

"You can take all the Aricept you want, but it isn't working."

The Only Way to Get Apoaequorin is Prevagen

I was curious about how Mark Underwood regarded the role of diet in Alzheimer's. Could you eat more of certain foods and get your necessary supply of apoaequorin?

"No food contains apoaequorin. Prevagen is the only way to get it. It's now made in a controlled scientific process, so no jellyfish are harmed."

"A lot of things have advanced in medicine by looking to a solution in nature," he continued. "Thirty years ago, we had to go to pigs for insulin. Now here we have a brain issue. We found something in nature from jellyfish that provides that benefit."

"Until we made the breakthrough, there was nothing to be done about the calcium problem, even though we knew about calcium."

Of course, many people with Alzheimer's or memory issues are on multiple medications. Is Prevagen safe for them?

"There are no problems with interactions with medicines," Mark told me. "You already have this protein in your body. It's always been safe."

Reduce Memory Errors by An Average of 19%

According to Prevagen's manufacturers, a large double blind, placebo-controlled trial called the Madison Memory Study was completed this year. 218 people were tested using a computer-based testing protocol developed by Cogstate, the world's leading cognitive testing software development company. The study confirmed actual changes in brain function in Prevagen users.

Among the significant findings, Prevagen was able to reduce memory errors by an average of 19%, compared to a placebo. The participants with the fewest memory problems saw an even greater improvement, underscoring the importance of being proactive when it comes to brain function.

Carolyn Got Back Her Confidence and Zest for Living

Now that Mark Underwood had explained the science, I wanted to talk to people who take Prevagen. What was their experience like?

Mark had already told me of a huge practical benefit that some Prevagen users have experienced. "We find individuals who were incontinent can now go to the bathroom again.

Their bladder was functionally fine. The problem stemmed from their brain. That makes a big difference in quality of life."

What else could Prevagen do? Through Mark's office, I got the names of two people with stories to tell about Prevagen. I had long talks on the phone with both of them, and I'd like to share their stories with you.

First, I spoke to Joan Snow, who's the caregiver to her father. Joan's father is now in his *ninth* year of Alzheimer's, and still living independently. He mows the lawn, fixes his own coffee, and keeps track of his pills. And since 2008, one of those pills is a daily dose of Prevagen.

"Two times, we've run out of Prevagen, and he's noticeably deteriorated without it," Joan told me.

"When he was off the Prevagen, my father couldn't remember my brother was there. My brother went 'Whoaaaaa.' He was shocked."

"My sister is skeptical of supplements, but she saw the bad effects when he was off it. She told me, 'You know, that's really doing something for Dad. And then, when I got him back on Prevagen, he went back to being himself. He didn't have that confusion."

As I listened to Joan Snow explain in detail how she manages her father's Alzheimer's, I was filled with admiration. I think Joan represents the gold standard in loving and attentive care.

In fact, I was so impressed with Joan that I decided to write a whole chapter about the nutritional and supplemental routine she's created for her father. You'll meet her in Chapter 11 and learn more about how she's helping to keep her father living in cheerful independence, as he approaches a decade of Alzheimer's.

In the meantime, I want to introduce you to 73-year-old Carolyn, who's been diagnosed with Alzheimer's. As Carolyn tells me her remarkable story, she speaks with the lovely lilt of her native South.

"I'm so active, but for some time I could feel myself slipping," Carolyn told me, when I asked how she'd been affected by Alzheimer's. "I'd leave the kitchen and walk to the bedroom and forget why. It would aggravate me. It's little stuff. I'd go to pour a pitcher of tea with my little spout and spill some. It sounds dumb, but I'd never done that before. It was something in my brain that made me lose track of what I was doing."

"We have plants, and I've actually killed some of them by watering them two or three times a day. I just didn't remember that I'd watered them."

"My husband didn't think that anything was wrong. But then he saw me in church. Since I was a little girl, I've won every Bible drill. I know that book! But then the pastor would ask us to turn to a passage, and I couldn't find my place in my Bible. When my husband saw me bumbling with my Bible, he said, 'Carolyn, we're going to the doctor.'"

"That's when I knew what kind of trouble I was in. I got goose bumps!"

"I went to the neurologist and told him that I'm having problems with my short-term memory. He examined me and said that I had early-stage Alzheimer's. I asked him, what's the most natural thing that can be done for me."

"He said, I don't know about that. I prescribe Aricept. He told me to take one a day. And then, he'd check me when he got back to town in six weeks."

"That night, I called my dear friend, Glenda, who's a private duty nurse in homes. She's worked with people with Alzheimer's. I asked her opinion of Aricept. She told me in her experience, the dosages have to keep being increased. She said, the patient I'm nursing now has gone from 5 mg of Aricept to 25 mg."

"And then Glenda told me, 'Carolyn, go online and get Prevagen.' Glenda told me that she knows of a family that put their mother in a nursing home. The daughter came, and stayed locally, and saw the goings-on in the nursing home. She was so unnerved that her mother didn't recognize her that she went out to Walgreens and bought Prevagen. She started going to the nursing home for breakfast and dinner and giving her mother Prevagen with both meals. Three weeks later, she brought her mom out of the nursing home. Mom knew her and the grandchildren. She completely raised up her mother's quality of life."

"Well, I took Glenda's advice and ordered the Prevagen. I only took the Aricept for seven days. On the eighth day, I stopped the Aricept. And, instead, I started taking the Prevagen. By the second week, I just started feeling a huge difference."

"We have a lunch we go to at the senior center, and I was always late. I'd set alarms and everything, but I didn't hear them. I didn't have a clue. All of a sudden, I was noticing it was almost noon, and I'd get there on time."

"I started remembering to put on the coffee at night, so it would be ready in the morning. Things like that. When the doctor came back in town, he talked to me for a long time and said, 'I'm just amazed. You're doing remarkably well. Usually, Aricept doesn't work that quickly.'

"I took out my bottles of Aricept and Prevagen and showed them to him. I said, I just took seven Aricept. See, you can look in the bottle; here are the rest of them. But I do take something else twice a day. It's called Prevagen."

"The doctor hadn't heard of Prevagen. I was so afraid that he would frown on this natural stuff. But he said, I've got a lot of patients that need to be on that. And he started reading back to me my test scores from last time. He said, the first three questions I tested you on before you got one out of three. Then one out four."

"This time you got *two* out of three and *three* out of four! Now if you were on the Aricept, I'd have to have you come every few weeks and do lab work on you to see if it affects your liver. But I've moved on to Plan B. I really think you're on to something."

"I told him I could cry happy tears. My husband has already commented that he's noticed the difference. He's a big sight-seer, and I'd gotten withdrawn and didn't want to do anything. I'd say to him, Honey, if you want to go see where Abe Lincoln lived, go right ahead. I'll wait in the car."

"Now I've started getting up at six in the morning. I've got so much energy, and I don't feel depressed. Now that I'm doing so well mentally, I'm actually over-active. My husband said I've started so many projects, he's afraid I'll overdo it."

"I pride myself on being alert and clear-thinking and helping people. And I'd gotten to where I couldn't make decisions. I just wasn't thinking right, and that's worse than any disease."

"Now I've got my good attitude back. I really don't think you have to lose your mind before you die."

Sources

www.prevagen.com

Interviews with Mark Underwood, Joan Snow, Carolyn, and Dr. Fred Pescatore

Chapter 4

Meet Dr. Fred Pescatore: "Decline is Not Inevitable"

Dr. Fred Pescatore must be one of the busiest men in New York. He's the President of the International and American Association of Clinical Nutritionists, and the director of a bustling medical center in Manhattan.

He's the author of the *New York Times* bestselling book, *The Hamptons Diet* and the #1 bestselling children's health book, *Feed Your Kids Well*. Dr. Pescatore's other books include: *Thin For Good*, *The Allergy and Asthma Cure*, *The Hamptons Diet Cookbook* and *Boost Your Health with Bacteria*.

Prior to opening his own practice, Dr. Pescatore was the Associate Medical Director of The Atkins Center for Complementary Medicine, where he worked closely with the late Dr. Robert Atkins.

Dr. Pescatore is a traditionally trained physician who has chosen to practice Integrative Medicine. For over two decades, Dr. Pescatore has treated patients with a combination of traditional and alternative medical techniques.

I was delighted that Dr. Pescatore found time in his action-packed day to talk with me. I began by asking him what goes through his mind when he first sees a patient with Alzheimer's. How does he begin to approach the problem?

"Whether it's Alzheimer's or Parkinson's or another condition, I approach patients from a diet and nutrition perspective," he answered.

"So I begin by looking at nutritional status. What are their levels of **zinc, magnesium, potassium, chromium, manganese**, etc.? Do they have sufficient **trace minerals**?"

"Then I look at their levels of **CoEnzyme Q-10**, which is very important. I also assess levels of **Vitamin A, Vitamin D, Vitamin B12** and **folic acid**."

"Next, I look at their diet. I recommend a low inflammation diet. That means eliminating sugar and simple carbs. You need to eat primarily proteins and vegetables, with some complex grains."

"I also do food sensitivity testing. Are they gluten intolerant? Do they have milk intolerance? Are there yeast issues?"

"I get them set on that part first. Then, number two, I recommend supplements that I've found work."

Healing Supplements that Boost the Brain

"For Alzheimer's, I recommend **gingko 120 MG three times per day, Vitamin A 10,000 IU twice per day and Vitamin D 5,000 IU per day,** and **NAC 1,000 MG twice per day**."

"In addition, I recommend **pycnogenol 100 MG twice per day**. Pycnogenol is a French maritime pine tree extract that supports blood flow to the brain."

"I also suggest **Prevagen, 10 MG per day**. The studies are really good on the jellyfish protein's ability to work on brain function."

"And there's a mushroom called **Lion's Mane** that's specifically formulated for brain issues, dementia, Alzheimer's. I recommend **500 MG twice per day**. There's good clinical research on it."

"The last thing I use is **NADH, 10 to 290 MG** in the morning. The brand name is **Enada.** It's in every brain cell and our bodies get depleted of it. It's used a lot in Europe."

"Some of these supplements are available through our website."

I'll go into detail about many of Dr. Pescatore's supplement recommendations in other chapters. You'll learn much more about their brain-boosting properties and the science behind their effectiveness.

I think you're going to be greatly encouraged by the healing powers of these woefully under-reported supplements. So keep reading!

He's Back to Doing the *New York Times* Crossword Puzzle!

Dr. Pescatore described for me the kind of transformation that such an integrative medical approach can spark.

"One man came in here, recently. His wife brought him in after a neurologist diagnosed him with Alzheimer's. He was a typical high-functioning New York guy and he was losing it. He couldn't focus. What really shook him up was that he couldn't do the *New York Times* crossword puzzle anymore, and that was important to him."

"Now he comes bouncing in here. His wife says he's back to his old self. He's even doing the crossword puzzle again."

Keep Trying and Don't Give Up

"I think people get put into categories where conventional medicine doesn't have anything to offer them. Unfortunately, I'm seeing too many people come here with regular dementia, not Alzheimer's, who have been put on Aricept. And there's no study for Aricept and dementia. There's no reason they should be put on that drug."

"From my perspective, there's always more you can try for Alzheimer's. For instance, I might try a homeopathic spray. I'd make sure their adrenal glands are working."

"Don't give up. Decline is not inevitable, even with an Alzheimer's diagnosis. Keep trying!"

For Further Information:

Dr. Fred Pescatore, 369 Lexington Ave., 19th Floor, New York 10017
Phone: 212 779-2944
Fax: 212 779-2941
Email: medicine369@yahoo.com
www.drpescatore.com
Dr. Pescatore offers a number of vitamins and other supplements on his website.

Chapter 5

Lion's Mane, the Medicinal Mushroom that Energizes Brain Neurons

"You will have nerves of steel and the memory of a lion." With those encouraging words, herbalists in ancient China would feed the emperor precious morsels of Lion's Mane.

I hope the emperor enjoyed his tasty tidbits of this medicinal mushroom, because he was the only one allowed to eat it: that's how highly prized Lion's Mane was throughout ancient Asia.

According to traditional Chinese medicine, Lion's Mane mushroom, or *Hericium erinaceus*, is a tonic of the highest order, capable of gently soothing the stomach and powerfully stimulating the mind. These ancient healers believed Lion's Mane could cure ulcers of the digestive tract and even heal cancers of **the esophagus, stomach and duodenum.**

Today, we're learning much more about the potential of this weird-looking mushroom with long white tendrils to combat Alzheimer's and dementia. Studies in Japan and China have probed its ability to stimulate re-growth in neurons, and to protect cells from toxic amyloid b, which forms the deadly protein plaques in brains afflicted with Alzheimer's.

As noted in the previous chapter, Dr. Fred Pescatore recommends Lion's Mane mushroom to his Alzheimer's patients, based on his assessment of clinical research that investigated Lion's Mane's effect on the brain.

Before I show you the clinical studies, you'll want to hear the incredible story of <u>why</u> Lion's Mane can help regenerate brain neurons.

How Young Rita Levi-Montalcini Dodged Bombs and Bullets to Discover NGF

The story begins with a determined young woman of unquestioned genius, hard at work in the makeshift laboratory she had just created in her bedroom. The year was 1940, and Dr. Rita Levi-Montalcini, a new medical school graduate in Turin, Italy, was eager to pursue her research in neurology.

But Fascist laws forbade Italian Jews from practicing medicine, so she improvised a lab at home. When bombs started falling, she fled to the countryside and rebuilt her lab in a cottage.

The burning question that drove Dr. Levi-Montalcini was how nerves emerge from an embryo's developing spinal cord and then branch into its budding limbs. In the war-torn countryside, she bicycled to farms to buy fertilized eggs for her experiments. Food was so scarce that after she finished her research on the eggs, she ate them.

After the war, Dr. Levi-Montalcini accepted an invitation at Washington University in St. Louis. There, she continued her groundbreaking research on nerve development.

And, in 1986, she won the Nobel Prize for medicine with Stanley Cohen for their discovery of nerve growth factor (NGF), a protein that causes developing cells to grow by stimulating surrounding tissue.

Here's what her official biography at Washington University states: "Their research, conducted in the 1950s, while members of the faculty of Washington University, is of fundamental importance to the understanding of cell and organ growth and plays a significant role in understanding cancers and diseases such as Alzheimer's and Parkinson's."

Alzheimer's Brains Lack NGF

As we age, our levels of NGF decline. And in people with Alzheimer's, the loss of NGF is catastrophic. Pietro Calissano, a collaborator of Dr. Levi-Montalcini, explained about NGF, "At the start, it seemed this molecule's effect was restricted to acting on the peripheral nervous system, but then it emerged that it has a very important role in the brain. Contrary to what was believed, the brain does not have a rigid structure but is in continuous movement, and NGF helps neurons – which we begin to lose between 10 and 15 years old – survive."

The horrible dilemma of treating Alzheimer's is that the brain needs more NGF…but it can't get it. The NGF protein molecule is too big to pass through the blood-brain barrier. Only small, fatty-like molecules can slip through this protective membrane. Designed to prevent foreign objects and harmful chemicals from damaging the brain, the blood-brain barrier also frustrates healing compounds from coming to the rescue by locking them out.

At least one major pharmaceutical company is striving to develop a drug that can deliver NGF to treat Alzheimer's. In 2008, Ceregene, Inc. announced that the University of California, San Diego had received a $5.4 million grant from the National Institute of Aging at the National Institutes of Health (NIH) to support a Phase 2 clinical study of Ceregene's CERE-110, a gene therapy product designed to deliver NGF for the treatment of Alzheimer's.

But here's the cold, hard fact: Ceregene's gene therapy product may or may not work. And even if it is successful, it probably will be many years before it comes on market.

However, in the meantime, there is a way to stimulate NGF production in the brain – and it comes from a mushroom!

Lion's Mane Can Help Stimulate NGF

It turns out that the Lion's Mane mushroom contains a bevy of bioactive compounds that can stimulate the production of NGF in the brain. How? Their low molecular weight allows them to sneak through the blood-brain barrier, and slip inside the brain!

And once inside, they can get to work, encouraging the production of NGF. Dr. Hirokazu Kawagishi of Shizoka University in Japan is the leading authority on Lion's Mane. Dr. Kawagishi and his team isolated a type of molecule in Lion's Mane called **hericenones** – *the very first active substance found in natural products that induces synthesis of NGF*!

Hericenones comes from the fruiting body of the mushroom, which sprouts out of the ground or tree. Dr. Kawagishi also discovered **erinacines**, another molecular compound found within Lion Mane's root system. And erinacines turn out to be even <u>more</u> robust at promoting NGF production.

Here's what Dr. Kawagishi and his colleagues wrote about the amazing potency of erinacines: "The newly-discovered erinacine H stimulated 31.5 /- 1.7 pg/ml of NGF secretion into the medium at 33.3 [micro]g/ml concentration, which was five times greater than NGF secretion in the absence of the compound. **The erinacines are the most powerful inducers of NGF synthesis among all currently identified natural compounds.**"

Dr. Kawagishi described the effects of Lion's Mane on patients in a study conducted in a rehabilitative hospital in the Gunma prefecture in Japan. The study followed 50 patients in an experimental group and 50 patients used as a control: "All patients were elderly and suffered from cerebrovascular disease, degenerative orthopedic disease, Parkinson's disease, spinocerebellar degeneration, diabetic neuropathy, spinal cord injury, or disuse syndrome. Seven of the patients in the experimental group suffered from different types of dementia."

"The patients in this group received 5 g of dried Lion's Mane mushroom per day in their soup for a 6-month period. All patients were evaluated before and after the treatment period for their Functional Independence Measure (FIM), which is a measure of independence in physical capabilities (eating, dressing, walking, etc.) and in perceptual capacities (understanding, communication, memory, etc.).

"The results of this preliminary study show that after six months of taking Lion's Mane mushroom, six out of seven dementia patients demonstrated improvements in their perceptual capacities, and all seven had improvements in their overall FIM score."

These results were borne out in another Japanese study, published in the journal *Phytotherapy Research* in March 2009. In this double-blind, placebo-controlled clinical trial, 30 Japanese men who were diagnosed with mild cognitive impairment were randomly divided into two 15-person groups. One group was given Lion's Mane, and the other given a placebo. The subjects of the Lion Mane's group took four 250 mg tablets containing 96% of Lion's Mane dry powder three times a day for 16 weeks. After termination of the intake, the subjects were observed for the next 4 weeks.

At weeks 8, 12 and 16 of the trial, the Lion's Mane group showed significantly increased scores on the cognitive function scale compared with the placebo group. The Lion Mane's group's scores increased with the duration of intake, but at week 4 after the termination of the 16 weeks intake, the scores decreased significantly. Laboratory tests showed no adverse effect of Lion's Mane. The study's researchers concluded that Lion's Mane "is effective in improving mild cognitive impairment."

Meet the Mushroom Guru

Lion's Mane is available in several brands, and I noticed that one of them is formulated by Paul Stamets. Stamets is an interesting character, a sort of Indiana Jones-like mushroom hunter who brings unmatched expertise to his forays throughout the old-growth forests of the Pacific Northwest.

Stamets calls himself a "Mycelium Messenger" – mycelia are the vegetative parts of a fungus – and he's dedicated thirty years to penetrating and protecting the astounding world of mushrooms. He's discovered four new species, invented numerous methods of cultivation, and written six books.

Stamets gives lectures on "6 Ways That Mushrooms Can Save the World," inspiring audiences with his vision of mushrooms that clean up toxins, revitalize ecosystems and cure a host of diseases.

And he's a big fan of Lion's Mane, which he says, "is nature's nutrients for your neurons."

Stamets has created a product line of mushrooms called Fungi Perfecti. You can buy his formulation of Lion's Mane through his website at www.fungi.com. He offers Lion's Mane in both capsule and liquid extract form.

Here's his description of his Lion's Mane capsules:

"This beautiful species, appearing as a white waterfall of cascading icicles, is found on broad leaf trees and logs. The subject of recent studies on nerve regeneration, Lion's Mane *(Hericium erinaceus)* is renowned for providing support to the brain and nervous system. Each capsule contains 500 mg of freeze-dried Lion's Mane mycelium. Available in bottles of 60 capsules."

As for dosage, Dr. Fred Pescatore recommends that Alzheimer's patients take **500 MG twice per day**.

If you want to consider another brand, here's a noteworthy option.

Amyloban Protects Against Toxic Brain Plaque

A Japanese research team isolated an additional compound from Lion's Mane called amyloban, which they patented. Their studies indicate that amyloban protects neurons from amyloid b, the toxic protein that forms the dangerous sticky plaque on Alzheimer's brains.

A company called Mushroom Wisdom produces both a proprietary brand of Lion's Mane and a separate supplement of amyloban, named Amyloban 3399.

Here's how they describe Amyloban 3399 on their website:

"Amyloid is a protein that may accumulate between the nerve cells (neurons) in the brain as we age. Amyloban® 3399 contains a proprietary extract from Lion's Mane (*Hericium erinaceus*) shown to support the survival of nerve cells in the presence of toxic amyloid (Japanese patent 394,3399, US patent pending). It also contains other active compounds (hericenones) from Lion's Mane that can stimulate the production of Nerve Growth Factor (NGF) in the brain.* Amyloban® 3399 was developed by the Mushroom Wisdom research team in collaboration with leading university researchers in Japan and China."

You can order Mushroom Wisdom's formulations of Lion's Mane and Amyloban 3399 through their website at www.mushroomwisdom.com

Be Smarter Than Ever at 102!

As you seek to renew your brain neurons with the NGF-promoting compounds of Lion's Mane, draw inspiration from the astonishing woman who first discovered NGF.

As of this writing, Dr. Rita Levi-Montalcini is 102 and still going to work every day at her laboratory in Italy, as immaculately dressed as ever.

She's the longest-living Nobel laureate of all time and still looking forward to the future. At her 100th birthday party celebration, she proclaimed, "At 100, I have a mind that is superior - thanks to experience - than when I was 20."

How does she do it? Pietro Calissano, who has collaborated with Dr. Levi-Montalcini, says that NGF may be stimulating her vitality. "Every day, she takes NGF in the form of eye drops," he said, "but I can't say for sure if this is her secret."

Sources:

www.fungi.com

www.mushroomwisdom.com

Ceregene
http://www.ceregene.com/science_alzheimers.asp

"Improving effects of the mushroom Yamabushitake (Hericium erinaceus) on mild cognitive impairment: a double-blind placebo-controlled clinical trial."
Mori K, Inatomi S, Ouchi K, Azumi Y, Tuchida T.
Mushroom Laboratory, Hokuto Corporation, 800-8, Shimokomazawa, Nagano, 381-0008, Japan. morikou@mail2.pharm.tohoku.ac.jp
John Wiley & Sons 2008
http://www.ncbi.nlm.nih.gov/pubmed/18844328

Townsend Letter for Doctors and Patients April, 2004
"The Anti-Dementia effect of Lion's Mane mushroom and its clinical application - Hericium erinaceus - Lion's Mane"
by Hirokazu Kawagishi, Cun Zhuang, Ellen Shnidman
http://findarticles.com/p/articles/mi_m0ISW/is_249/ai_114820665/?tag=content;col1

Ultimate Immune.com
"Lion's Mane: Neural Nourishment"
http://www.ultimateimmune.com/articles/lions-mane.php

On Dr. Rita Levi-Montalcini:
Nature
"One Hundred Years of Rita"
By Alison Abbott
April 1, 2009
http://www.nature.com/news/2009/090401/full/458564a.html

The Independent
"Is This the Secret of Eternal Life?"
Peter Popham
April 25, 2009
http://www.independent.co.uk/news/science/is-this-the-secret-of-eternal-life-1674005.html

Washington University School of Medicine
Women in Health Sciences
http://beckerexhibits.wustl.edu/mowihsp/bios/levi_montalcini.htm

Huffington Post
"Rita Levi Montalcini, Nobel Prize-Winning Scientist Turns 100, Still Works"
April 18, 2009
http://www.huffingtonpost.com/2009/04/20/rita-levi-montalcini-nobe_n_188935.html

Chapter 6

Tracking Down the Amazing, Elusive Methylene Blue

Join me now as I play detective in a high-stakes mystery drama. The outcome could have real impact on Alzheimer's patients and their families, so stay with me through the story's surprising twists and turns.

In the summer of 2008, two news stories rocked the world of Alzheimer's research. First, in July, the *London Times* splashed a headline proclaiming, *"New drug Rember brings 'unprecedented' Alzheimer's treatment advance."*

Then, in August, *Science Daily* trumpeted *"Potential Alzheimer's, Parkinson's Cure Found in Century-Old Drug,"* in an attention-grabbing story on methylene blue.

The claims made for both **Rember** and **methylene blue** were so extraordinary that online Alzheimer's chat rooms buzzed with anticipation and hope. When my research uncovered them, I was plenty excited, too.

Rember was described by its scientific team at the University of Aberdeen as slowing Alzheimer's progression *by up to 81%,* and proving at least twice as effective as current medications, such as Aricept.

"The most significant development" since Alois Alzheimer's discovery in 1907

Professor Claude Wischik and his colleagues focused on 321 Alzheimer's patients in Britain and Singapore, dividing them into four groups. Three groups took varying doses of Rember; the fourth took a placebo.

The group that took a 60mg dose of Rember for 50 weeks showed an 81% reduction in mental decline compared with the placebo group.

So how did Rember work?

Professor Wischik's study demonstrated that Rember successfully targeted the neurofibrillary tangles that characterize Alzheimer's. "This is the most significant development in the treatment of the tangles since Alois Alzheimer discovered them in 1907," Professor Wischik said.

The *Times* article quoted Dorothie Hardie, whose 72-year-old husband had participated in the study. "Two years ago, if Jimmy had gone to his shed he may have forgotten what he was about to do. Now he is able to plan, get the tools he needs and do the task."

"We appear to be bringing the worst affected parts of the brain functionally back to life," Professor Wischik said, as quoted in the *Daily Mail*.

"It is the first realistic evidence that a new drug can improve cognition in people with Alzheimer's," said Professor Clive Ballard, head of research at the Alzheimer's Society in England.

Where's Rember Now? The Trail Goes Cold

A follow-up article in the *London Times* reported that the patients who had received Rember during the trial were worried about stopping the drug. But Professor Wischik said he would try to continue to supply them with Rember on a compassionate basis.

But what about everybody else who desperately wanted to try it? After the initial *Times* article appeared, Alzheimer's patients and their families besieged Professor Wischik, begging to join his next trial.

I tried to track down Rember, but the trail went cold. It takes years for a promising drug to come to market, and Rember seemed to be lost in endless bureaucratic proceedings.

All the hope, all that excitement…and no way to get to it. How sad!

I turned my attention to the other drug that made headlines in 2008 as a potential Alzheimer's cure, methylene blue.

A Cheap "Wonder Drug" for the Brain Named Methylene Blue

But finding methylene blue proved to be equally vexing.

Science Daily reported that a study conducted by researchers at Children's Hospital & Research Oakland had achieved highly promising results with low doses of methylene blue.

Microscopic amounts halted cellular aging in mice and boosted their mitochondrial function, particularly of a crucial enzyme called complex IV. Mitochondria are the powerhouses of the cell, providing energy.

"One of the key aspects of Alzheimer's disease is mitochondrial dysfunction specifically complex IV dysfunction, which methylene blue improves," said Dr. Hani Atamna, the head researcher. "Our findings indicate the methylene blue, by enhancing mitochondrial function, expands the mitochondrial reserve of the brain. Adequate mitochondrial reserve is essential for preventing age-related disorders such as Alzheimer's disease."

Dr. Atamna's colleague, Dr. Bruce Ames, added, "What we potentially have is a wonder drug."

But where was it? Methylene blue was supposed to be a century-old, common and inexpensive drug. But I kept hitting brick walls, trying to track it down.

And I noticed people in Alzheimer's chat rooms were trying to find it, too. In fact, I read an online discussion about the possibility of buying a bottle of it from an aquarium supply shop and diluting it to use as medicine.

Let me quickly cut to the chase about that option: DON'T DO IT! Unless you don't mind swallowing the cyanide that goes along with it.

As a matter of fact, don't even try to hunt down methylene blue on your own.

Now, getting back to our story, I must admit I was getting mighty frustrated. Locating both Rember and methylene blue was proving to be unexpectedly difficult.

And then, I discovered something that absolutely floored me…

Rember *is* Methylene Blue!

When I interviewed Dr. Jacob Teitelbaum, the renowned physician, author, and chronic fatigue syndrome expert, he startled me by saying that he recommends methylene blue as a possible option for Alzheimer's.

Methylene blue, he explained, is "old as dirt. It's cheap and non-patentable. So it's not out there making billions as an Alzheimer's treatment, as it should."

"But a drug company could try to patent the delivery system, which is what Rember is."

Wait! So Rember is essentially a dressed-up version of methylene blue?

"That's right. Although it will be 4-5 years before the FDA process for Rember is completed, so it can be approved for Alzheimer's and available in pharmacies, the optimal dose is 60 mg 3 x day (more is not better)."

"In the meantime, methylene blue can be prescribed by holistic physicians and made by compounding pharmacies."

Then Dr. Teitelbaum revealed a weird fact: *taking methylene blue will turn your urine blue.* That's because methylene blue is a dye that gets excreted in the urine.

I asked Dr. Teitelbaum to recommend a compounding pharmacy that would provide methylene blue, and he gave me the following information. He also emphasized that you shouldn't try to find it on your own.

Where to Get Methylene Blue

Dr. Teitelbaum recommended Cape Apothecary of Annapolis, Maryland, and its pharmacist, Dr. Thomas J. Wilson.

I called Dr. Wilson and spoke to him, and he said that he'd be happy to compound methylene blue and ship it to you, providing you have a prescription.

"Methylene blue may have a hard time proving itself in studies, because it turns urine blue," Dr. Wilson said, when I asked him for his thoughts about it. "You can't test against a placebo, because people know they're taking it. There's no hiding it because of the urine color."

"It's certainly not going to harm a patient, as opposed to Aricept and Namenda. They can cause problems."

"We've done it several times and had no problems. Patients did well on it."

Here's the contact information for Cape Apothecary and Dr. Thomas Wilson:

http://capedrugs.com/
1384 Cape Saint Claire Rd. Annapolis, MD 21409
Contact Us
410-757-3522 410-974-1788 1-800-248-5978
Fax: 410-626-7226
drtomw@capedrugs.com

A Warning for Patients on Psychiatric Medications

In July 2011, the FDA issued a warning that it had received reports of serious central nervous reactions when methylene blue was given to patients taking psychiatric medications that work through the serotonin system of the brain (serotonergic psychiatric medications).

They recommend that patients taking **serotonergic drugs** not take methylene blue, unless necessary for life-threatening treatment, such as cyanide poisoning.

Sources:

Interviews with Dr. Jacob Teitelbaum and Dr. Thomas Wilson

London Times
"New drug Rember brings 'unprecedented' Alzheimer's treatment advance"
July 30, 2008

London Times
"Rember, the drug that helps Alzheimer's sufferers"
August 3, 2008

Daily Mail
"Daily pill that halts Alzheimer's is hailed as 'biggest breakthrough against disease for 100 years"
By Jenny Hope
July 29 2008
http://www.dailymail.co.uk/health/article-1039677/Daily-pill-halts-Alzheimers-hailed-biggest-breakthrough-disease-100-years.html

Drugs.com
"Methylene blue: Drug Safety Communication – Serious CNS Reactions Possible when given to patients taking certain psychiatric medications"
July 26, 2011

Science Daily
"Potential Alzheimer's, Parkinson's Cure Found in Century-Old Drug"
August 18, 2008
http://www.sciencedaily.com/releases/2008/08/080818101335.htm

Endfatigue.com
"Alzheimer's and Senility are Reversible"
by Dr. Jacob Teitelbaum
http://www.endfatigue.com/health_articles_a-b/Alzheimers-and_senility_are_reversible.html

Chapter 7

Increase Blood Flow to the Brain with Pycnogenol, a Pine Bark Extract

I first heard about Pycnogenol as an Alzheimer's supplement from Dr. Fred Pescatore. "It's a French maritime tree extract that supports blood flow to the brain," Dr. Pescatore explained. "Any time you have damage to tissue, increasing blood flow is an important treatment modality."

"And Pycnogenol has been the subject of over 200 studies, confirming its safety and efficacy."

Considering that your brain requires 20 percent of your body's oxygen, and that it suffers huge harm from decreased blood supply, Pycnogenol's power to deliver blood to the brain sounds like a very good thing.

Pycnogenol is the brand name for an herbal supplement extracted from the bark of the French maritime pine tree. Its source is a coastal forest of millions of acres in Southwest France, near the famous Bordeaux region.

When I think of southern France, I picture beautiful vineyards and rolling hills. From now on, I'll also imagine big pine trees growing for fifty years, tended without pesticides or herbicides, and brimming with active chemical compounds that nourish the brain.

Australian Researchers Find "Significant" Cognitive Improvements

In July 2008, researchers from Swinburne University in Australia published an exciting study in the Journal of Psychopharmacology. 101 elderly participants (60-85 years) had consumed a daily dose of 150 mg of Pycnogenol for a three-month treatment period.

The study, which used a double-blind, placebo-controlled, matched-pair design, found that the Pycnogenol group displayed "statistically significant" improvements in memory scores, relative to the control group.

Not only that, the Pycnogenol group had markedly lower concentrations of biomarkers for oxidative stress and damage from free radicals!

And what works for seniors seems to help younger minds, too. An Italian study conducted at Pescara University proved that college students who took Pycnogenol for eight weeks showed notable improvements in alertness, memory and mood.

Dr. Gianni Belcaro's research team randomly assigned 108 Italian university students to receive either a daily 100 mg dose of Pycnogenol or placebo for eight weeks. Computer-measured results indicated that the Pycnogenol group showed improvements in attention, memory and mood, *while levels of anxiety decreased by 17%!*

"More interestingly, in this study the cognitive performance of the subjects was evaluated in a real challenging situation like the university examinations," wrote Dr. Belcaro in a 2011 article in the journal Panminerva Medica.

Dr. Belcaro stated that Pycnogenol's benefits may be linked to its ability to boost blood circulation and provide antioxidant protection.

Bioflavonoids to the Rescue, Reducing Inflammation

As the research makes increasingly clear, Pycnogenol's pine bark contains a unique combination of bioflavonoids, procyanidins and organic acids that offer a bonanza of health benefits.

Together, these nutrients can act as a powerful anti-inflammatory agent. And that's good news for Alzheimer's sufferers whose brains are marred by significant inflammation.

How does Pycnogenol work? According to the *Journal of Inflammation*, pine bark extract shuts off naturally occurring enzymes associated with inflammatory conditions.

Nutrition expert Jack Challem is a big fan of Pycnogenol and in his book, *The Inflammation Syndrome*, he explains why. While visiting the British Museum in London, Challem tripped and seriously injured his right foot.

The pain persisted for weeks, and he grew increasingly worried that he'd suffered a permanent injury. "And then it dawned on me," wrote Challem. He remembered that at a recent conference, he'd heard about Pycnogenol and its potent anti-inflammatory effects.

"I started taking it, and within days the pain went away. To rule out the power of suggestion, I stopped taking the supplement for a few days, and the pain returned. I started taking the supplement again and the inflammation and pain went away and have never returned. I walk and hike long distances without any discomfort in the foot."

How New World Explorers Got Cured from A Deadly Disease

Although Pycnogenol is gaining increased attention now, the rejuvenating power of pine bark has been cherished for centuries by native healers.

In 1535, French explorer Jacques Cartier and his crew became ice-bound in present-day Canada. Many of the sailors contracted scurvy, a deadly disease induced by lack of Vitamin C. In his journal, Cartier wrote that, "out of 110 that we were, not ten were well enough to help the others, a pitiful thing to see."

After 25 crew members died, the local natives helped to nurse the survivors back to health with teas and other concoctions made from tree bark. An entire tree was used up in less than a week, as the natives struggled to save the Frenchmen from the brink of death. Astounded by his crew's rapid recovery, Jacques Cartier wrote in his journals that the tree bark was a miracle sent by God.

Now the story skips ahead 400 years to Dr. Jacques Masquelier, a renowned French pharmacist and researcher. In 1951, Dr. Masquelier read Cartier's journal entries about his crew's miraculous recovery, and decided to find the medicinal compounds in the healing tea.

Eventually, Dr. Masquelier discovered the maritime pine tree and succeeded in extracting a chemical compound from its bark. He patented his process and dubbed his extract Pycnogenol.

Berkeley Scientist Discovers Super-strength Antioxidant

Today, researchers use cutting-edge science to probe the intricacies of pine bark's powers. And, increasingly, its restorative effects seem to have direct relevance to the problems of Alzheimer's.

You already know that Pycnogenol enhances blood flow and that Alzheimer's brains suffer from decreased blood supply. You also know that Pycnogenol has anti-inflammatory effects, and that Alzheimer's is a disease of inflammation.

So now let's turn to Pycnogenol's status as a super-strength antioxidant. Antioxidants are chemicals that deactivate free radicals and halt their cellular rampages. Like other degenerative brain diseases, Alzheimer's is characterized by oxidative damage caused by free radicals. And that's where Pycnogenol's superb antioxidant talents come in to the picture.

Let's meet Professor Lester Packer, who's widely regarded as the world's foremost antioxidant research scientist. Dr. Packer received his Ph.D. in Microbiology and Biochemistry from Yale University and headed the Department of Molecular and Cell Biology at the University of California, Berkeley for many years. Dr. Packer also established a laboratory in the Department of Molecular Pharmacology & Toxicology at the University of Southern California to study molecular, cellular, and physiological aspects of free radical and antioxidant metabolisms in biological systems.

And here's what Dr. Packer and his Berkeley team discovered, according to a Berkeley press release:

"An extract of pine bark has proven to be one of the most potent antioxidants, a property that may explain why pine bark has been used in folk medicine around the world, according to a new report by scientists at the University of California, Berkeley."

"Lester Packer and his colleagues at UC Berkeley screened many natural compounds for antioxidant activity and found that pine bark extract, marketed as Pycnogenol (trademark) (pik-nah-je-nal), is the most potent of the lot."

"In the past year and a half, Packer and his colleagues have documented a number of strong antioxidant effects of Pycnogenol that place it among the most potent antioxidants, ranking with vitamins E and C, and lipoic acid."

"Packer also recently found that Pycnogenol extends the lifetime of vitamin C in the body, prolonging its beneficial effects as an antioxidant."

(In a later chapter, you'll read about vitamin C and E and their dramatic partnership in neutralizing free radicals and protecting against Alzheimer's. So Pycnogenol's capacity to boost vitamin C certainly does catch my interest.)

Here's what Dr. Packer said about it:

"We looked at extract of fruits and vegetables, gingko, green tea and many other plants, as well as purified flavonoids, and among these Pycnogenol was the most potent in extending the lifetime of the vitamin C radical."

"There may be many flavonoids in Pycnogenol that affect the antioxidant network by interacting at the level of vitamin C. This helps to explain how pine bark extract has a beneficial effect."

UC Berkeley also reported that, "Packer has proposed a complex network of interaction between vitamin E, vitamin C (ascorbate) and other chemicals that effectively recycle those potent antioxidants and extend their effect in the body. Flavonoids like those in Pycnogenol seem to insinuate themselves into the network to help recycle E and C and extend their lifetimes even more."

Pine Bark Extract Fights off "Sticky Plaque" of Alzheimer's Brains

A leading cause of Alzheimer's brain damage is the protein amyloid b, which forms a sticky plaque that attaches to the brain and kills off cells. Dr. Benjamin Lau and his colleagues at Loma Linda University in California investigated Pycnogenol's ability to prevent damage caused by amyloid b.

Dr. Lau's team discovered that Pycnogenol helps to prevent amyloid b from inflicting vascular damage. When Pycnogenol was present, blood vessel cells successfully fended off amyloid b toxicity.

Dr. Lau also tested the memory of older mice who were regularly fed Pycnogenol. They showed markedly improved memory and learning ability in comparison to their littermates without Pycnogenol. And older mice treated with Pycnogenol for two months retained memory levels almost equal to those of young mice. Other researchers who carried out related studies with an extract of Gingko biloba had to feed 10 to 20 times as much to mice.

Moreover, in an eye-opening study, Dr. Dave Schubert of the Salk Institute in La Jolla, California investigated Pycnogenol's effect on neurons. And Dr. Schubert discovered that Pycnogenol helps to prevent neuronal cells from amyloid b-induced damage!

Dosage and Safety Guidelines

You can buy Pycnogenol in your local drugstore, health food store, pharmacy, or on the Internet. You'll find dozens of different brands and formulas to choose from.

Jack Challem, author of *The Inflammation Syndrome*, recommends Solgar's 100-mg Pycnogenol capsules. Solgar's website notes that its Pycnogenol capsules are vegetarian and kosher.

Dr. Fred Pescatore recommends that Alzheimer's patients take 100-mg of Pycnogenol twice a day.

Pycnogenol is generally considered safe, but there are some advisories.

If you have "auto-immune diseases" such as multiple sclerosis (MS), lupus (systemic lupus erythematosus, SLE), rheumatoid arthritis (RA), or other conditions: Pycnogenol seems to increase the immune system. By increasing the immune system, pycnogenol might decrease the effectiveness of medications that decrease the immune system. If you have one of these conditions, it's best to avoid using Pycnogenol.

Medications that decrease the immune system include azathioprine (Imuran), basiliximab (Simulect), cyclosporine (Neoral, Sandimmune), daclizumab (Zenapax), muromonab-CD3 (OKT3, Orthoclone OKT3), mycophenolate (CellCept), tacrolimus (FK506, Prograf), sirolimus (Rapamune), prednisone (Deltasone, Orasone), corticosteroids (glucocorticoids), and others.

If you take **Coumadin** or other blood thinning medications, be careful, because Pycnogenol could thin the blood.

Mild Pycnogenol side effects could include nausea, headache, or dizziness. You may want to consider starting with Pycnogenol 30 mg a day, and then working up to a higher dosage.

Sources:

Pycnogenol.com
http://pycnogenol.com/media/media_about.php

Journal of Psychopharmacology
"An examination of the effects of the antioxidant Pycnogenol® on cognitive performance, serum lipid profile, endocrinological and oxidative stress biomarkers in an elderly population"
July 2008 vol. 22 no. 5 553-562
http://jop.sagepub.com/content/22/5/553.abstract

Anabolic Minds
"Pycnogenol Improves Brain Function"
Stephen Daniells
December 8, 2011
http://anabolicminds.com/forum/content/pycnogenol-improves-brain-775/

Source: *Panminerva Medica*
2011, Volume 53, Supplement 1 to No. 3, Pages 75-82
"Pycnogenol supplementation improves cognitive function, attention and mental performance in students"
Authors: R. Luzzi, G. Belcaro, C. Zulli, M. R. Cesarone, U. Cornelli, M. Dugall, M. Hosoi, B. Feragallo

About.com
"Pycnogenol - Natural Pain Relief for Osteoarthritis"
By Carol Eustice
December 17, 2009
http://osteoarthritis.about.com/od/alternativetreatments/a/pycnogenol.htm

University of California, Berkeley
"Pine bark extract is a potent antioxidant, and may help boost the effects of vitamin C and other antioxidants, UC Berkeley scientists report"
by Robert Sanders
February 5, 1998
http://berkeley.edu/news/media/releases/98legacy/02_05_98a.html

Medline Plus
U.S. National Library of Medicine

http://www.nlm.nih.gov/medlineplus/druginfo/natural/1019.html

Smart Publications
"Pine Bark Extract: The Superb Antioxidant for Healthy Circulation"
http://www.smart-publications.com/articles/pine-bark-extract-the-superb-antioxidant-for-healthy-circulation/page-3

The Inflammation Syndrome
By Jack Challem
John Wiley & Sons, 2010

Interview with Dr. Fred Pescatore

Chapter 8

Meet Dr. Ronald Hoffman:
"Be Optimistic and Innovative"

Dr. Ronald Hoffman is one of the pioneers of complementary and alternative medicine. In 1985, he established the Hoffman Center as one of New York's first comprehensive practices for the delivery of innovative medical care. Today, Dr. Hoffman serves as Medical Director of the Hoffman Center, focusing on what he calls Intelligent Medicine: the concerted deployment of rational conventional medical strategies, side by side with nutrition, herbs, vitamins, and supplements.

Dr. Hoffman has served as president of the country's largest organization of complementary and alternative doctors, the American College for Advancement in Medicine (ACAM). After receiving his Bachelor's Degree from Columbia College and his M.D. from Albert Einstein College of Medicine, Dr. Hoffman attended the Tristate School of Traditional Chinese Medicine.

Dr. Hoffman is eager to share his knowledge of Intelligent Medicine with the widest possible audience. He hosts a popular, nationally syndicated radio program called "Health Talk," and is the author of several books, including *How to Talk with Your Doctor* and *Natural Cures that Really Work*.

I was intrigued to know what goes through Dr. Hoffman's mind when a patient comes in with signs of memory loss and dementia. How does he approach the medical challenges of Alzheimer's?

"I think one of the big elements in reversing cognitive decline is getting people off of unnecessary medications that have a brain-stultifying effect," he told me, in a fascinating phone interview. "Keeping them on statins and sleeping pills and medicines for blood pressure and other common conditions can really have a negative effect on their cognitive function."

"Are any of these medicines absolutely essential for preserving life? Because what I see is that people light up when they go off of them."

"And, very often, they really energize with B12 shots. B12 is vitally important in maintaining the health of nerve cells. If you have B12 deficiencies, your energy and concentration are going to be sapped. And your levels of homocysteine, which is a risk factor for circulatory disease, are going to dangerously rise."

"**Vitamin B12** deficiencies can be quite common in the elderly, due to malabsorption of food or lack of hydrochloric acid. If a patient hasn't been properly diagnosed with Vitamin B12 deficiency, we can really light somebody up with a series of injections. They perk right up."

"And then there are supplements that can help. For instance, **CoEnzyme Q10** for brain function is important. So is **DHA fish oil**, which has a brain-preserving effect. There's a lot of evidence that **Huperzine A (Chinese moss)** helps with mild cognitive decline. **Curcumin** is also very good. **Vitamin D** is essential. Alzheimer's patients are all low in Vitamin D, and taking them outside won't do it in the winter. **DHEA** has brain effects in both sexes. **Melatonin** is good for the sundowning symptom of Alzheimer's, in which patients become agitated in the late afternoon through evening."

"Grandma Is Now Sharp As A Tack!"

"Three months ago, I had a case that illustrates these points. A family brought in their 88-year-old grandmother, who had been a university professor. She was confused and experiencing memory loss and cognitive decline."

"When I saw her, she was obviously overmedicated. We took her off of her unnecessary medications. We also discovered that she had gluten sensitivity and vitamin B12 deficiencies. We addressed all these issues, through dietary changes and a series of shots. And we recommended a program of supplements."

"Well, she has turned around dramatically. The family told me, 'She's now sharp as a tack. We've got grandma back!'"

"You do have to have a support system for this kind of program. I had a case of a woman who came to me with Alzheimer's. She arrived late by herself, and told me that her granddaughter was downstairs watching the car. I said, 'I'm not going to charge you for today, because I can't see you alone. You need someone to be with you.'"

"I insist on a family commitment. We see some amazing families with such cohesion. But it does require structure and encouragement."

"For instance, Alzheimer's patients need to be on a Type 3 Diabetes diet. That means giving people ultra-high protein, low carb diets with lots of fat. I recommend using **coconut oil, avocados, and full fat dairy products**.

"**Whey protein shakes**, which are a building block of glutathione, with **fresh blueberry** are very good. That would be an excellent lunch for an Alzheimer's patient."

"And it's important that Alzheimer's patients reduce their sugar. Alzheimer's is a catabolic state, in which people become emaciated and lose muscle mass. Often they have taste disturbances and crave sugar. And some medicines can make you crave sugars, too."

The Supplemental Regimen that Woke Up E.K.'s Mind

On Dr. Hoffman's website, he tells the story of E.K., an Alzheimer's patient treated at his center. At age 73, E.K. developed memory lapses, crying every morning, believing her parents were alive. She began getting lost while going out alone, and accusing family members of stealing her things. By the time Dr. Hoffman saw her three years later, E.K. had even begun to forget her family. She could remember her name, but almost nothing else.

Dr. Hoffman gave E.K. a series of B12 shots 3 times weekly for two weeks, then started her on monthly injections. She was put on a gluten-free diet. And he placed her on a combined regimen of nutritional supplements, which were faithfully administered to her by her son.

Here is E.K.'s supplemental regimen:

• Multivitamin

• Vitamin E 800 IU

• Folate 5 mg

• B6 25 mg

• Vitamin C 4 gms

• Inositol 12gms

• DHEA 25mg

• Thiamine 400 mg

• Alpha-lipoic acid 2000 mg

• Acetyl-L-carnitine 1000 mg

• DHA (Docosahexaenoic acid) 1000 mg

• Ginkgo Biloba extract 320 mg

• NADH 10 mg

• N-acetylcysteine 200 mg

• Phosphatidylserine 300 mg

Dr. Hoffman reports that E.K. gradually and steadily improved to a remarkable degree. Her family first noticed that she was calmer and her sleeping pattern had reverted to normal. She no longer had panic attacks when left alone, and she was able to dress, bathe and eat independently.

After two years, her neurologist noted these huge improvements in an insurance report: "Patient seems to have recovered significant memory over the last two years from natural process/or the employment of vitamin supplements in collaboration with family members. Improvement has been seen especially in areas of ADL (Activities of Daily Living), i.e. independence in self dressing, eating and light cooking. There is absolutely no issue about continence. There is no evidence of sleep-wake cycle, mood changes, agitation, wandering or other affective or personality disorders. She has reached a stable plateau in her neurological state with no evidence of progressive deterioration. I would presently classify her as having minimal dementia in the order of Age Related Memory Loss."

Be Optimistic and Take an Innovative Approach

As Dr. Hoffman acknowledges in his written commentary on this case, it's unclear exactly which component of this regimen produced such a positive outcome. "But the essence of targeted nutritional therapy is the synergy between diverse agents simultaneously addressing multiple regenerative pathways." In other words, you can't know exactly what element is working, but if the combination produces results, keep doing it.

As we close our conversation, Dr. Hoffman tells me, "I believe in taking an innovative approach. I don't think we've solved the problems yet, but we can mitigate and ameliorate the symptoms. We've kept people alive longer, and they've felt happier and calmer. They've had time to enjoy life and spend time with their grandchildren. I'm an optimist."

Further Information:

http://www.drhoffman.com/
The Hoffman Center
776 Sixth Avenue
Suite 4B
New York, New York 10001

The Center: (212)779-1744
The Store (for supplemental products): (800)456-9384
Fax: (212)779-0891
TheHoffmanCenter@aol.com
Dr. Hoffman has created supplemental brain-health products that you can buy through his website.

Chapter 9

P.S. I Love You:
Discover PS, The Essential Fatty Nutrient That Erases 12 Years From the Brain

Before I tell you the inspiring story of how former Pentagon researcher Nita Scoggan rescued her husband Bill from advanced Alzheimer's, I want to ask a question.

Why don't more people know about the extraordinary memory-boosting powers of phosphatidylserine (PS)?

It's been researched many times. More than 35 human studies attest to its vital role in memory and cognitive function. 16 clinical trials have detailed PS's ability to restore memory and ramp up learning, vocabulary, and concentration – all mental activities linked to age-related decline.

And that's not all. PS is such a blessing for the brain that it can even beat the blues. People suffering from depression perk up with PS, and feel more engaged, happy, and sociable.

Most famously, Dr. Thomas Crook proved that *PS can make the brain act 12 to 14 years younger*!

Dr. Crook was an internationally recognized memory expert who conducted extensive research on just about every drug designed to treat Age Associated Memory Impairment (AAMI). For fourteen years, he worked at the National Institute of Mental Health where he served as Chief of the Geriatric Psychopharmacology Program.

And here's what he said about PS: **"PS is by far the best of all drugs and nutritional supplements we have ever tested for retarding AAMI."**

Consider the astounding results of a study Dr. Crook conducted at Stanford and Vanderbilt Universities, and in his research clinics in Maryland and Arizona. 149 men and women with age-related memory impairment were either given 300 mg of PS daily or a placebo for twelve weeks. At regular intervals, they were assessed for learning, attention, and memory.

After just *three weeks* of treatment, the group taking PS scored significantly higher at key memory skills such as remembering names and telephone numbers, memorizing paragraphs, and locating objects like glasses and keys.

And after twelve weeks, PS had restored the ability to remember names by 14 years… and to learn and recall written information by 12 years!

So let's return to our question: Why don't more people know about PS?

No Money for Pharmaceutical Companies in PS

In a revealing 2005 interview, Dr. Crook commented, "Since PS is not protected by patent, there is little incentive for companies to fund further research when existing data can support claims related to memory. If a pharmaceutical company had proprietary rights to PS we could do some very interesting studies, but that is not the case."

In other words, the big money is in expensive prescription drugs that may not be as effective and may, in fact, inflict harm.

No wonder the big companies can't patent PS: it's a naturally occurring substance in your body. PS is a phospholipid, a class of fatty nutrients that maintains healthy cell membranes and speeds transmission of messages between brain cells.

Since PS is a naturally occurring substance in the body, it's considered quite safe as a supplement. "There are no reported drug, nutritional supplement, food, or herbal interactions with phosphatidylserine," wrote Marwan Sabbagh, M.D. in his book, *The Alzheimer's Answer*.

PS Keeps Brain Cell Membranes Healthy and Flexible

Your body manufactures PS, but can also access it from eggs and organ meats. However, lots of people have been scared off of eating eggs. And these days, organ meats are not exactly a popular item in the average person's diet.

That means you've got to rely on your own internal production of PS. And as you get older, your ability to manufacture it can often drop significantly.

Without sufficient PS, brain cell membranes grow rigid, and neurons falter in their communication. Energy production also sputters, because PS plays a major role in fueling brain cells.

The result? Confusion, brain fog, memory loss, depression, and mental decline.

How Phosphatidylserine Gave Bill Scoggan His Brain Back

Nita Scoggan was desperate. After four years on Aricept, her beloved husband Bill was rapidly sliding downhill into advanced Alzheimer's.

He couldn't dress himself. He had no idea where the bathroom or kitchen was in his own house. He didn't want to get out of bed. In fact, he could barely speak.

But Nita just knew that somewhere inside this passive shell of a man was the brilliant dynamo she had married. During a long, successful career in Washington, D.C., Bill Scoggan had held high-level jobs at the Pentagon, with responsibility for over 100 employees.

And yet, here he was, helpless as a child, unable to even feed himself. Worse yet, he was becoming increasingly aggressive and potentially violent.

The doctors told Nita to send him to a nursing home and prepare herself for his imminent death. But Nita, guided by her religious faith, refused to give up on Bill. Determined to use the skills she'd honed as a Pentagon researcher, she delved into reading everything she could about Alzheimer's.

In 2003, she stumbled upon PS in her investigations, and decided to give it a try. Encouraged by European studies that showed PS's benefits for patients with severe dementia, Nita began giving Bill 100 mgs of PS, three times a day for a month.

And then she began to track his behavior. The first month, she didn't see any real change. But at the beginning of the second month, a small incident occurred that jolted her with excitement and hope.

She said to Bill, "Honey, I'm going to get the cereal." And Bill responded, "I'll get the bowl." *And then he stood up and got it*!

He was talking; he was moving; he was aware of what was going on and he knew where to find things!

It was stunning. And that was only the beginning. Shortly thereafter, Nita was watching "Who Wants to Be A Millionaire" on television…and Bill began shouting out the answers!

Encouraged by Bill's stirrings of life, Nita boosted his dosage of PS, eventually reaching 1,000 mg a day. And Bill continued to get better…and better…and better.

The Doctor Was Drop-Jawed at Bill's Miraculous Recovery

When Nita took Bill to the Veterans Administration doctor, he was flabbergasted. "Whatever you're doing, keep it up," he said. "Bill is doing great."

For a year, Nita kept Bill on both the Aricept and PS, as Bill's mental functioning, strength, and liveliness returned. Then she decided to drop the Aricept and rely on PS.

And to her delight, Bill kept steadily improving. He functioned with complete independence; not only could he feed himself, he could also cook!

Astoundingly, he began cutting the lawn with a power mower – something he hadn't been capable of for *ten years*!

When Nita took Bill for his annual exam, the doctor's jaw dropped. "His recovery is nothing short of a miracle," said the doctor.

And then Nita confessed…She had taken Bill off of the Aricept a full year ago. The miracle the doctor was witnessing with his own eyes was due to the healing powers of PS.

"I hope you'll recommend it to your patients," Nita said.

"I'd lose my license if I did," the doctor replied.

Alzheimer's Defeated! Daughter Wins Her Mom Back!

Today, Nita and Bill Scoggan try to get out the word about their remarkable experience with PS. They give radio and television interviews, available on YouTube, which you'll find charming and inspiring.

And Nita has written a book called *Boost Your Brain Digest*, available through her website, in which she shares her hard-won knowledge about restoring brain health.

On her website, (www.nitascoggan.com) Nita offers advice to families grappling with Alzheimer's. She urges patience, because you may not get instant gratification at the start of PS supplementation.

Sometimes, you can see greater energy and enhanced function within days or a couple of weeks. But often, it takes a few months for enough PS to accumulate within the brain to stimulate a noticeable improvement. And the more advanced the Alzheimer's, the longer it may take for the improvement to kick in.

Getting a sufficient dosage to spark recovery can also make the difference.

On Nita's website, she features a letter written to her, under the stirring headline: **"Alzheimer's Defeated! Daughter Wins Her Mom Back!"** In it, a daughter writes about seeing Nita and Bill on television, and deciding to try PS supplementation on her mother, who had grown "confused and hostile."

She began giving her mother 100 mg of PS a day, but her mother continued to deteriorate. Then she read Nita's book, and decided to increase the PS to 1000 mg a day. But even with the much greater dose, her mother showed no improvement.

Desperate, she raised her mother's PS dosage to 1600 mgs a day, and kept on, hoping against hope, for three months. And that turned the tide!

Her mother's memory came back, her appetite increased, and she started engaging in conversations.

In June, the daughter lowered the dose to 1200 mg a day, as her mother's improvement continued. In October, she lowered it to 900 mg daily, and in December, she decreased it to 600 mg a day.

And her mother got better every step of the way!

"She is alert and aware of her surroundings. Mom has started doing things for herself – brushing her teeth, feeding herself, saying her prayers, putting her gloves on. She knows her birthday again. She will soon begin physical therapy. I will continue to give her 600-900mg of PS daily in her applesauce, I know Mom will keep on improving."

So What's the Right Dosage of PS?

Dr. Ronald Hoffman's regimen for Alzheimer's includes 300 mg of PS daily. Nita Scoggan recommends 300 mg as the minimum amount. Higher doses may be called for if the progression of the disease is advanced.

Nita recommends soft gel caps, which are available in the chain store GNC. As a practical matter, she suggests that if the patient has trouble swallowing, you can open the soft gels and stir the contents into food or put it in a milk shake.

And here's her most important advice of all: *Be encouraged! Don't give up*!

Sources:
Nita Scoggan's website:
www.nitascoggan.com

Whole Foods Magazine
"Phosphatidylserine and the Memory Cure"

"An Interview with Thomas H. Crook III, Ph.D."
by Richard A. Passwater, Ph.D.
September, 2005
http://www.drpasswater.com/nutrition_library/Nov_05/Crook_PS_Edit_a.html

The Better Brain Book

David Perlmutter, M.D., FACN and Carol Colman

Riverhead Books, 2004

The Alzheimer's Answer

Marwan Sabbagh, M.D.

John Wiley & Sons, 2008

The Alzheimer's Prevention Plan

Patrick Holford with Shane Heaton and Deborah Colson

Piatkus Books, 2005

Chapter 10

Huperzine A, the Plant Extract the Chinese use to treat Alzheimer's

What's the most widely used treatment for Alzheimer's in China? If you guessed "huperzine A," you've obviously been cracking open the latest issues of *Cell Biochemistry and Biophysics!*

Huperzine A is a health-giving, alkaloid compound extracted from the legendary Chinese moss plant (*Huperzia serrata*). For thousands of years, the Chinese have treasured huperzine A for its gentle healing of fever and inflammation.

And now, inspired by eye-popping clinical studies in China, leading American research labs are probing its astonishing potential to remedy Alzheimer's.

Works Like Aricept, but Better!

What particularly intrigues me is that huperzine A appears to work in strikingly similar fashion to many standard Alzheimer's prescription medications: Aricept (donepezil), Exelon (rivastigmine), Razadyne (galantamine), and Cognex (tacrine).

But the good news is that huperzine A may work better, safer and longer, with fewer, if any, side effects.

"Compared to the medication tacrine, huperzine A appears to cross the blood-brain barrier more readily, remain effective longer, and have less potential for the development of drug tolerance and liver toxicity," wrote Dr. Rallie McAllister, a board-certified family physician and author.

Dr. McAllister also noted that patients with Alzheimer's and dementia who take daily supplements of huperzine A "experience significant gains in terms of mood, memory, behavior, overall clinical status and quality of life."

Patients don't just think better; they also feel better and enjoy increased mobility.

So how does huperzine A work? Well, it turns out that both huperzine A and the standard prescription drugs mentioned above are acetylcholinesterase (AChE) inhibitors. They work by suppressing the enzyme AChE, a major villain in the Alzheimer's drama.

The nastily destructive AChE breaks down acetylcholine, a vitally needed chemical messenger in the brain. Acetylcholine allows your brain to perform its normal functions of learning, thinking and memory.

If you've got Alzheimer's, chances are good that acetylcholine-producing neurons in your brain have been damaged or killed off, and that you're running seriously short of enough acetylcholine for healthy brain function.

By taking huperzine A, you can help stomp out the destructive enzyme AChE, so it doesn't destroy the scant supply of acetylcholine that you've got left.

The Chinese Studies That Excited American Scientists

Starting in the 1980s, Chinese scientists discovered that huperzine A substantially improves memory and cognitive function in patients with Alzheimer's and other forms of dementia.

Excited by this new use of a millennia-old remedy, they began conducting a series of major studies on huperzine A's effect on the brain.

In 2002, a Chinese research team randomly divided 202 Alzheimer's patients into two groups. One set took huperzine A 400 micro g/day for 12 weeks; the other ingested a placebo. Incredibly, *59% of the huperzine A group showed notable improvement in behavior and mood,* and raised their cognitive scores by 4.6 points!

And in 2008, a research team at China's Sichuan University reviewed the results of six clinical trials of a total of 454 Alzheimer's patients. Once again, by significant margins, huperzine A stimulated improvements in memory and cognitive function.

More recently, in 2011, *Cell Biochemistry and Biophysics* published the results of a new double-blind, placebo-controlled study in China that examined the effect of huperzine A in patients with mild to moderate vascular dementia.

Patients who took daily supplements of huperzine A for 12 weeks showed big boosts in their cognitive scores and in their abilities to perform activities of daily living, compared with those taking a placebo of vitamin C.

The Natural Way to Fight Brain Plaque and Protect Nerve Cells

Huperzine A has quite a few other superhero powers.

It's a terrific **antioxidant**, fighting back against oxidative stress caused by free radicals in the brain. Alzheimer's is associated with increased oxidation of lipid, protein and DNA molecules.

That's why it's potentially hugely important news that a Chinese clinical study showed that patients taking huperzine A experienced major reductions in blood markers of oxidative stress.

It **protects against the death of nerve cells in the brain** that are linked to Alzheimer's. This nerve damage is spurred by abnormal activity of glutamate, a neurotransmitter that can incite neurons to fire out of control.

Are you taking **Namenda,** a commonly prescribed drug for Alzheimer's? Namenda is the brand name of **memantine,** one of a class of drugs that performs this same function of protecting nerve cells from out-of-control glutamate. These drugs are known as NMDA receptor antagonists.

Unfortunately, memantine was just found to be ineffective for mild Alzheimer's. And its list of possible side effects is downright bloodcurdling: extreme tiredness, dizziness, confusion, back pain, headache, vomiting, shortness of breath and hallucination!

The day may be coming when huperzine A is widely acknowledged as getting the job done in a gentler, safer, more effective way than memantine.

Huperzine A wards off **brain plaque damage.** One of the defining characteristics of Alzheimer's is sticky plaques. Made of beta-amyloid protein, they form on blood vessels and nerve cells in the brain. A huge benefit to Alzheimer's patients could be huperzine A's protective properties against beta-amyloid.

Focus, Memory, Concentration and More

XEL Pharmaceuticals is developing a once-a-week huperzine A patch, which they say will promote better absorption and more reliable blood levels. Their commitment to this product stems from their studies of huperzine A's abundant health benefits, which they list as the following:

What are the Benefits of Huperzine A?

• Treatment of Alzheimer's Disease

• Treatment of vascular dementia

• Treatment of cognitive and memory impairment

• Learning and memory retention

• Improved focus and concentration

• Improved nerve transmission to muscles

• Powerful and reversible long-term inhibitor of AChE activity in the brain

- Dementia resulting from strokes and senile or presenile dementia

- Improved clinical picture for patients with myasthenia gravis

- Improved short-term and long-term memory in patients with cerebral arteriosclerosis (hardening of arteries in the brain)

- Alleviation of symptoms related to glaucoma

- Prevention of organophosphate pesticide toxicity

- Prevention of nerve gas toxicity

Breakthrough at Yale Could Change Medical History

Leading American research labs have taken note of the Chinese studies on huperzine A, and are enthusiastically delving into research, too.

Dr. Paul Aisen, professor of neurology at Georgetown University Medical Center's Memory Disorders Program, designed a major study at 23 locations in 12 states, examining huperzine A's impact on Alzheimer's.

Dr. Paul Aisen said, "Based on studies in China, huperzine A may be more effective and better tolerated than currently prescribed drugs for Alzheimer's disease. In addition, laboratory studies suggest that huperzine A may have unique effects that could slow down the progression of the disease… trial is essential to better understand the promise of huperzine A."

And now, there's news of a gigantic breakthrough at Yale University.

Extracting huperzine A from the Chinese moss plant has always been a painfully slow, difficult business.

But Dr. Seth Herzon led a research team that has devised a completely new method of creating huperzine A that is quick and cost-effective. He published his findings in the August 25, 2011 issue of the journal *Chemical Science*.

"Being able to synthesize large amounts of huperzine A in the lab is crucial because the plant itself, which has been used in Chinese folk medicine for centuries, takes decades to grow and is nearing extinction due to overharvesting," said Dr. Seth Herzon.

Dr. Herzon's team created an eight-step procedure to process huperzine A that has the potential to drive down the cost from $1,000 per milligram to just 50 cents.

The U.S. Army is backing Dr. Herzon's research, because they're interested in its apparent capacity to counter chemical warfare agents, without side effects.

Dr. Herzon is working on producing huperzine A on an industrial scale and bringing its healing to legions of Alzheimer's sufferers. He notes that huperzine A works similarly to current prescription medications for Alzheimer's, but it binds better, lasts longer and is more easily absorbed.

"We believe huperzine A has the potential to treat a range of neurologic disorders more effectively than the current options available," Herzon said. "And we now have a route to huperzine A that rivals nature's pathway."

Dosage and Caveats for Taking Huperzine A

Huperzine A hasn't yet penetrated mainstream medicine. Most doctors happily write a prescription for Aricept, or another standard AChE inhibitor, without giving a single thought to huperzine A, even though it may perform the same function better and more safely.

But a lot of natural-minded doctors know about huperzine A and recommend it to their Alzheimer's patients. Among them is Dr. Ronald Hoffman, who told me that he considers it well-studied for its improvements on mild cognitive impairment and Alzheimer's.

Dr. Hoffman makes a formula that includes huperzine A called Advanced Brain Sharp, which you can buy on his website (www.drhoffman.com). Huperzine A can also be purchased separately.

According to Beth Israel Deaconess Medical Center, the recommended daily dose is **100 to 200 micrograms** twice a day for age-related memory loss. They advise that you use it only under a doctor's supervision.

Occasionally, huperzine A causes mild side effects like dizziness, nausea and diarrhea, which usually diminish over time. It's not known to adversely affect vital signs like blood pressure or pulse.

But if you're taking prescription AChE inhibitors already, like Aricept or Cognex, it's not a good idea to take huperzine A, too. No need to overdo it.

Sources:

Interview with Dr. Ronald Hoffman

Your Health by Dr. Rallie McAllister
"Herbal Extract May Improve Brain Function in Alzheimer's Patients"
http://www.creators.com/health/rallie-mcallister-your-health/herbal-extract-may-improve-brain-function-in-alzheimer-s-patients.html

Alzheimer's Reading Room
"Scientists Create Natural Huperzine A, Alzheimer's Fighting Compound in Lab"
August 26, 2011
http://www.alzheimersreadingroom.com/2011/08/scientists-create-natural-huperzine.html

XEL Pharmaceuticals Huperzine A Transdermal Matrix Patch
http://xelpharmaceuticals.com/XEL001HP.php

EmaxHealth
"Natural Compound Huperzine A Fights Alzheimer's, Made in Lab"
by Deborah Mitchell
August 26, 2011
http://www.emaxhealth.com/1275/natural-compound-huperzine-fights-alzheimer's-made-lab

Beth Israel Deaconess Medical Center
"Huperzine A"
www.bidmc.org/YourHealth/ConditionsAZ.aspx?ChunkID=21761

The Alzheimer's Answer
Marwan Sabbagh, M.D.
John Wiley & Sons, 2008

Chapter 11

Hard-Won Wisdom from a Loving Caregiver

I was deeply moved by my talk with Joan Snow, and I think you will be, too. Joan embodies the power of love, coupled with a fierce determination to not give up on a family member with Alzheimer's. The results may amaze you, and give you new hope for prolonging and uplifting the lives of Alzheimer's patients.

Joan's 75-year-old father is now *nine* years into Alzheimer's and his doctors are stunned at his healthy condition. They say he should either be dead or imprisoned in a wheelchair, unable to understand what's going on around him.

Instead, he lives by himself. He mows the lawn and fixes his own coffee. He keeps track of his medicines. And, most important of all, he enjoys and appreciates life.

Joan's devotion to her father is heartwarming. She calls him every day. She visits him often and cooks him healthy meals. And she spends a lot of her free time on the Internet, researching Alzheimer's and learning about new supplements and remedies to help her father.

"My mom was the one who took care of Dad before she died," Joan explained to me. "She worried about his memory and took him to the doctor, who diagnosed him with Alzheimer's. They put Dad on Aricept, then they switched him to Namenda. In 2007, he got on the Exelon patch."

"Of course, there's a problem with the prescription drugs for Alzheimer's. If you read through their side effects, they're the same symptoms as Alzheimer's!"

"Mom began researching different supplements for Dad. She got him on **Juice Plus**, which is juice powder concentrates from 17 fruits, veggies and grains. She also got him on **curcumin** and **ALA (Alpha Lipoic Acid)**, which he still takes."

"Mom bore the brunt of the situation, because she was with him all the time. He often got depressed and moody."

"Then my mom got sick with pancreatic cancer and died in 2007. We were amazed that he stayed so steady after losing her. They were married almost fifty years. Well, Dad just took over her duties, doing the grocery shopping and laundry. He'd call me and say, 'How often do you change the sheets?' We were stunned."

"I began to spend my time researching Alzheimer's. I got him on **Prevagen**, and I started taking it. When I start him on something, I take it myself to see if there are side effects. He's run out of Prevagen twice and we all noticed that he deteriorates without it."

"I do the **coconut oil** for him. I like to make him smoothies with it. He also takes **fish oil** and **lithium orotate**. I've got him on **Total Recall**, a brain supplement by a company called Super Good Stuff. I'm wondering if I should up Dad's dosage of that."

"He's also on **grape seed extract**, which passes the blood brain barrier. He's on **ubiquinol**, which is a form of **Coenzyme Q10** that's more available to the body."

"He takes **Memeron**, which is a natural form of **galantamine**. That's derived from the snow lily."

"He also takes **Cerefolin**, a prescription drug for B vitamins. And he's on **probiotics** for bladder issues."

I asked Joan how her father keeps track of his medications. "He's an engineer," she replied. "Very methodical in his thinking. He's got an AM pill container and a PM pill container, and he figured out how to keep track. We fill them up two weeks at a time."

"His doctor says that after nine years of Alzheimer's, he should be in a home, needing full time care. He should not be able to recognize us. In fact, he should be reduced to saying one word."

"Instead, he lives on his own and takes care of the house and yard by himself. I try to call him every night, and see how he's doing. And I go over and make him some healthy meals that he can heat up, because I know my mom would be horrified at the thought of him eating frozen dinners."

"We've just passed the four year mark for losing my mom. His neurologist is still amazed and his test scores are about the same as they were in 2006, when he first started seeing him."

"You know, he was quiet when we were growing up, and not very sentimental. But now, he's so loving and appreciative. He hugs and kisses my sister and me all the time. He says, I don't know what I'd do without you girls. He's a sweetheart."

"We really believe that it's a miracle from God that he is doing so well."

Joan is lucky to still have her father, and her father is blessed to have Joan. I believe her commitment to his health has greatly enriched and extended his life. May they enjoy many more precious years together!

Chapter 12

Curcumin, the Miracle Spice that Protects Indians' Brains from Alzheimer's

What gives curry its beautiful orange color? The surprising answer is curcumin, a champion protector of brain function and one of the most highly prized fighters against Alzheimer's.

Curcumin is the active compound in the popular Indian spice turmeric, a main ingredient in many Indian dishes. Curcumin's anti-inflammatory powers are legendary, and so are its fantastic antioxidant properties.

Some researchers attribute the relative rarity of Alzheimer's in India to the frequent use of turmeric in the typical Indian's diet. "India has one-third the level of Alzheimer's that we do, and it's probably because of curcumin," Dr. Jacob Teitelbaum told me.

Many natural-minded doctors list curcumin as an essential supplement for Alzheimer's, including Dr. Teitelbaum and Dr. Ronald Hoffman.

In fact, Dr. Teitelbaum told me he considers curcumin the supreme supplement for Alzheimer's prevention. "If you're going to do something for prevention, take curcumin," he said. "It's probably the premiere herb for reducing the risk of Alzheimer's."

"The animal studies on it are pretty dramatic," he noted. "The curcumin actually melted the tangles in the brain."

And that's just what a crew of brilliant researchers in California discovered…

UCLA Scientists Prove Curcumin Breaks Up Brain Plaque

Scientists at the University of California Los Angeles made a huge breakthrough when they fed curcumin to elderly mice: *the plaques of beta-amyloid protein in the mice's brains actually disintegrated*! Those plaques, of course, are the hallmarks of Alzheimer's in humans.

Even better, when they added low doses of curcumin to <u>human</u> beta-amyloid proteins in a test tube, the curcumin did what some experts thought was impossible. It actually prevented the beta-amyloid proteins from combining and stopped cold the formation of damaging plaques.

Dr. Gregory Cole, the study's co-author wrote, "The new findings suggest that curcumin could be capable of both treating Alzheimer's and lowering a person's risk of developing the disease."

Even the mainstream is noticing that the ancient spice of curry may hold state-of-the-art medicinal relief.

New York Times Applauds Curcumin's Relief of Joint Pain

In October 2011, *The New York Times* ran an article titled *The Doctor's Remedy: Turmeric for Joint Pain*. It touted curcumin as a famous anti-inflammatory that relieves pain from achy joints.

The Times reporter interviewed Dr. Minerva Santos, director of integrative medicine at Northern Westchester Hospital, who proclaimed, "I use a lot of turmeric in my practice. It's an amazing spice."

The Times cited a recent study published in *The Journal of Alternative and Complementary Medicine*. Researchers found that curcumin was as powerful as ibuprofen in providing pain relief and improved function in 107 people with knee osteoarthritis.

In fact, curcumin is widely studied, with hundreds of published articles that investigate its exciting potential for cancer and its healthy effect on the cardiovascular system.

So why don't more people take curcumin?

Well, there's been a problem…

If It Stays In Your Gut, It Doesn't Enter Your Bloodstream

Curcumin is notoriously hard for the body to absorb. Dr. Santos explains that in India, people usually have pepper in their meal, which helps the curcumin enter the bloodstream.

You'd have to mix lots of pepper and curry and eat highly spicy food all day to get the curcumin you need. And the results wouldn't be optimal, anyway.

You want curcumin that's easy to ingest, a cinch for your body to absorb, and that stays in your bloodstream for hours as it brings constant anti-inflammatory relief to your brain.

And, according to Dr. Jacob Teitelbaum, that wasn't possible – till now.

CuraMed Is Absorbed Up to 10 Times Better Than Plain Curcumin

"Curcumin is difficult to absorb in the body," Dr. Teitelbaum said. "But now there's a new form of it called CuraMed that's made by EuroPharma. This company does very good work at optimizing absorption."

"Take one a day to prevent Alzheimer's. Take two a day if you have Alzheimer's. CuraMed is in a very easily absorbed form."

Dr. Teitelbaum is so enthused about CuraMed's absorbability that he put me in touch with Cheryl Myers, EuroPharma's Chief of Scientific Affairs and Education.

She wrote me the following letter, which I found filled with intriguing information:

Happy to help. I have attached a little info on some of the work being done using our CuraMed BCM-95 curcumin in the field of Alzheimer's. The abstract attached is on a 6-month study of AD patients examining serum markers of beta-amyloid destruction. It did not examine cognition or behavior. At Edith Cowen University, there is a study under way by Dr. Ralph Martins, a very prestigious AD researcher, that does look at cognition. He is comparing our BCM-95 curcumin to placebo in early stages of dementia to see if it will slow the progression of the disease, which is the expected outcome.

We are fortunate to participate in research such as this. The reason they choose to use our form of curcumin is because it is absorbed -- up to 10 times better than plain curcumin. That means they can give 2 or 3 capsules a day instead of 20 or 30. Also, it is maintained in a therapeutic range above 100 ng/g in the blood stream for 8 hours or more. Other forms of curcumin—even those with enhanced absorption—tend to shoot up and then down again, with levels above this mark lasting only 45 minutes to 2 hours. Lastly, our BCM-95 curcumin is not extracted with harsh solvents. We use only derivatives of alcohol and acetic acid (vinegar) to pull the curcumin from the turmeric rhizome. As the demand for and price of curcumin escalates, companies are starting to use class one (the most dangerous kind) petroleum-based solvents to try to extract curcumin from even poor quality turmeric. The residual of some of these solvents are neurotoxic. Our product has been shown to be safe and non-toxic, even at higher doses, in human studies.

I think you can tell I am pretty fond of our curcumin. I believe it is perhaps the most important plant medicinal under investigation today and can help so many people who have chronic illness, whether it is AD, or cancer, or arthritis, or heart disease—the list goes on.

Before I started working in the world of natural medicine, I worked a great deal with patients suffering from dementia—usually AD. I taught a course on differentiating dementias and dementia care at Tri-State University in Indiana, and served as secretary of the governor's older adults protective services team. I have seen first-hand the emotional pain and disability caused by this disease, so I have a special incentive to help people disseminate good information on how to best help these patients.

Best wishes,

Cheryl Myers
Chief of Scientific Affairs and Education
EuroPharma, Inc.

I was impressed with the credentials of Dr. Ralph Martins, who's conducting studies with CuraMed. Based in Australia, Dr. Martins is a longtime researcher into Alzheimer's, and a pioneer in isolating the beta-amyloid protein that forms the characteristic plaque deposits in the Alzheimer's brain.

Dr. Martins observed that clinical work with curcumin has required very high dosing in past studies, because of its absorption problems.

"I chose BCM-95 curcumin (CuraMed) for this human study because it has published bioavailability data. Therefore, I can use a reasonable amount and expect that the serum levels will achieve a therapeutic range for a significant period of time," Dr. Martins wrote.

Take Vitamin D3 with Curcumin to Enhance Alzheimer's Protection

Dr. Milan Fiala of UCLA has discovered how to get even more Alzheimer's-fighting capacity from curcumin: use it with Vitamin D3. His research revealed that taking Vitamin D3 with curcumin empowers the body's "clean up crew" to more efficiently remove the dangerous amyloid-beta protein from the brain.

"Vitamin D3 and curcumin offer new treatment possibilities for Alzheimer's," said Dr. Fiala.

The best way to get Vitamin D3 is to walk in the sun. Twenty minutes of striding outside in the natural sunshine is good for the heart, the soul, and the brain. But when the biting January winds blow, you can stay cozy indoors, eating Vitamin D3-rich cold-water fish (make sure you purchase a brand that's mercury-free), eggs and yogurt. You can also take a capsule supplement of Vitamin D3. For people over 50, the recommended dose is 10 mcg.

A Caution About Taking Curcumin if You're on Blood Thinners

If you're on a blood thinner like warfarin or Plavix, don't take curcumin without first consulting your doctor (hopefully, one who's receptive to nutritional medicine). Curcumin is a blood thinner itself. So are a number of other safe, proven supplements including proteolytic enzymes. Very likely a nutritional doctor can transition you from pharmaceutical blood thinners to natural ones like curcumin.

But in any event, because of curcumin's blood-thinning attributes, don't take it for at least two weeks before scheduled surgery.

Also, according to a recent *New York Times* article on turmeric and curcumin, it's advisable to steer clear of curcumin if you've got gallstones or problems with your gallbladder.

Sources:

Interview with Dr. Teitelbaum; letter from Cheryl Myers

Journal of Biological Chemistry

"Curcumin Inhibits Formation of Amyloid β Oligomers and Fibrils, Binds Plaques, and Reduces Amyloid *in Vivo*"

Fusheng Yang, Giselle P. Lim, Aynun N. Begun, Oliver J. Ubeda, Mychica R. Simmons, Surendra S. Ambegaokar, Pingping P. Chen, Rakez Kayed, Charles G. Glabe, Sally A. Frautschy, Gregory M. Cole
December 7, 2004
http://www.jbc.org/content/280/7/5892.abstract?sid=8c8b2e1b-d1f9-4ee1-a9f4-6cb766256a99#target-2

The New York Times
"The Doctor's Remedy: Turmeric for Joint Pain"
by Anahad O'Connor
October 19, 2011
http://well.blogs.nytimes.com/2011/10/19/the-doctors-remedy-turmeric-for-joint-pain/?src=me&ref=health

Natural Health Dossier
"Nature's Simple Combination to Prevent Alzheimer's"
August 12, 2011
www.naturalhealthdossier.com

EuroPharma – CuraMed
www.europharmausa.com/products/curamed-750-mg/

The Alzheimer's Prevention Plan
Patrick Holford with Shane Heaton and Deborah Colson
Piatkus Books, 2005

Chapter 13

Meet Dr. Jacob Teitelbaum:
"The Alzheimer's Just Goes Away"

Dr. Jacob Teitelbaum, M.D., has a remarkable story to tell. As a young medical student, he developed chronic fatigue syndrome/fibromyalgia and had to drop out of school. Eventually, he recovered enough to finish his studies and become a board-certified internist. In the ensuing 35 years, he's dedicated his career to developing effective treatment for fibromyalgia and other debilitating diseases.

Dr. Teitelbaum is the Medical Director of the national Fibromyalgia and Fatigue Centers and the author of the bestselling books *From Fatigued to Fantastic!, Pain Free 1-2-3, Beat Sugar Addiction NOW!*, and his most recent book, *Real Cause, Real Cure*.

A frequent guest on "Good Morning America," "The Dr. Oz Show" and other television shows, Dr. Teitelbaum lectures to patient, physician and research groups internationally. He is the lead author of groundbreaking "gold standard" research on effective treatment for chronic fatigue syndrome and fibromyalgia.

When Dr. Teitelbaum called me from his home in Hawaii to share his insights on Alzheimer's, I was quite startled by his uncompromising candor.

I was also intrigued by his pared-down approach to reversing Alzheimer's. Unlike some of the other doctors I interviewed, "Dr. T" places a premium on keeping things as simple as possible. For him, less is more, as far as supplements are concerned.

So brace yourself for some genuine shockers…

STUNNER: Half of People Diagnosed with Alzheimer's Don't Have It!

"The majority of people diagnosed with Alzheimer's don't have it," Dr. Teitelbaum said bluntly. "They have other problems that were missed. And those problems could have been treated!"

"Remember, the only way to diagnose Alzheimer's is with an autopsy. And a recent study of 426 autopsied brains in Hawaii showed about *half* of those diagnosed with Alzheimer's didn't have it. They lacked the toxic clumps and protein tangles that are the hallmarks of Alzheimer's."

"Dementia can have lots of different causes – and *many of them are treatable.* If you have low thyroid, vitamin deficiencies, low testosterone, poor sleep or depression, any of those can cause dementia. Even dehydration can cause dementia!"

"The problem is that most doctors don't have time to do a thorough evaluation for underlying causes. That would take about thirty to sixty minutes, and Medicare pays poorly for visits over five minutes."

"So what typically happens is that a family member is confused and gets taken to the doctor. Then, it's a matter of 'Round up the usual suspects. Grandma's got Alzheimer's. Here's a prescription.' But the prescription is hopelessly inadequate."

"Even if they do have Alzheimer's, you can do things that improve their brain function by that crucial five or ten percent. That's the difference between being independent or living in a nursing home. That's the difference between driving or not, and knowing who your kids are."

How To Tune Up Your Brain

"I tell people with Alzheimer's, let's give your brain a tune-up. When was the last time that you were functioning well? When were you driving and living on your own? Two years ago? Fine. Let's take you back to where you were two years ago."

"So how do you do a brain tune-up? Well, first, you optimize nutritional support. It's easy to give a really good multi-vitamin. I formulated a powder called **Energy Revitalization System** that's the equivalent of 35 pills in one drink. You take a scoop of the powder and add it to water. I recommend it for everyone over age 15. It also helps with diabetes and heart disease."

"Once they have the nutritional support they need, people start to feel a whole lot better on many levels. Now some people may experience loose stools from a powder. If they do, they can take a tablet multi-vitamin, instead. I recommend a brand called **My Favorite Multiple**."

"I'll note that if they take **Coumadin [a blood thinner]**, they can't take these multi-vitamins or ANY supplement without their physician's approval, so their blood test can be rechecked. For other medications, the interactions are generally not significant."

"Now for Alzheimer's patients or patients experiencing cognitive difficulties, I'd add one or two things to the multi-vitamin. A good **fish oil** is important. That's because the brain is made of DHA, the oil found in fish oil. A good choice is **Vectomega Oil**, a new Omega 3 source that comes from salmon brains (and fish is called brain food for a reason!). It's farmed from the fjords in Northern Europe, so you don't have mercury issues. And if you have hidden depression present, the fish oil can help with that, too. All it takes is 1-2 Vectomega a day, instead of 8-16 caps of most fish oils."

"I like to keep things simple. I don't like people taking handfuls of pills all day. Make it easy."

"I'd also add a third thing, which is optional. It's **ribose**, a health energy sugar. There's a brand called **Corvalen**. Take a 5 gm scoop of it and add it to the vitamin powder every morning."

"And then there's an herb that's probably the premiere herb for Alzheimer's prevention – **turmeric** or **curcumin**. The animal studies are pretty dramatic – it actually melted the brain tangles."

"It's difficult to absorb into the body, though. But now there's a new form of it called **CuraMed**. It's from a company called **EuroPharma** that does good work at optimizing absorption. Take two a day if you have Alzheimer's; one a day to prevent Alzheimer's."

What to Eat

"Now let's turn to the issue of diet. First, it's important to stay hydrated with water, not with sodas."

"And you should avoid excess sugar. You'll have more energy to shop and cook, and you'll experience fewer cravings without the sugar. Once you feel better and your brain works better, your junk food cravings will decrease."

"So go with a **high protein diet**. Eat **whole foods**. That means fruits, veggies, whole grains, lean meats, and fatty fish like salmon, tuna, mackerel, and herring."

"If convenient, it's preferable to choose lean meat without hormones or antibiotics. But I don't like to tell somebody who can barely button their blouse that they have to shop around for items that may be hard to find."

"Now, this first phase of getting the nutritional support in place can take two or three weeks. You usually see the beginnings of improvement by then. And six weeks should be a fair trial of how it's working."

Take A Holiday From Over-Medication

"Meanwhile, I'd be making arrangements with a doctor to try the next big picture item: seeing what medications the doctor can wean them off of. Which medications can they take a break from for a week to see if there's a side effect? Even just four or five days can help, to see if it's a drug that's causing confusion."

"When people get off of all these drugs, the results can be dramatic. People find their Alzheimer's goes away! Many elderly are on a mix of 10-15 medications! If you and I were on all these drugs, we'd be cross-eyed. The cops would be pulling us over for DUI."

"For instance, pain or depression medicines can cause brain fog, especially when you're combining them. It may be possible to see remarkable things when you're weaned off of many medications."

"Now your doctor may not want to do this. It's easy to write a new prescription; it takes 30 seconds. It takes much more time (and risk to the doctor) to stop a medication. And even if your regular doctor is well-meaning, this approach does take a lot more time, and the average doctor has four to six minutes per visit."

"So what should you do if your doctor has his head shoved up his rear? Go see another doctor! Get a good holistic doctor who will take the time to see what's going on with your medicines – and who's willing to help you wean off of those you may no longer need."

"To find a holistic doctor, you can go to www.holisticboard.org."

Experience the Healing Power of a Good Night's Sleep

"Now the next order of business is sleep. Are they getting less than seven hours a night? Being sleep-deprived contributes to confusion and loss of mental function."

"I suggest simple herbs. Take **magnesium** at bedtime, 200 to 400 mg. Some people get the runs from it. If you do, you can get **sustained released magnesium** from Jigsaw Health."

"If you need more help falling asleep, try **melatonin**, 1 mg at bedtime."

"And if you still need something else, there's an herbal mix called the **Revitalizing Sleep Formula** by Enzymatic Therapy. Take 1 – 4 capsules at bedtime."

"The herbal mix contains valerian. About 5% of people get energized by valerian. If you're one of them, don't take it. Do something else. Otherwise, this herbal mix is outstanding for most – without the risk of falling and confusion caused by too many sleeping pills."

"And avoid excessive caffeine. Do all these things, and you should be getting eight hours of sleep."

Take A Walk In The Sun

"Now you're well rested from sleep. You've got good nutritional support and you're not being over-medicated."

"You should have more energy. Go take a walk outside. Exercise and sunlight are good for you."

"The advice to avoid sunshine is insane! It increases the risk of falling and osteoporosis. Get out there and walk. The proper advice is to avoid sunburn."

Look for Hidden Infections and Hormonal Imbalance

"The next step is to look for hidden infections, especially of the bladder. Bladder infections are very common, and not all of them are symptomatic."

"Most bladder infections are caused by E. coli. You can knock it out with a supplement called **D-Mannose**. It's a simple sugar that occurs naturally in many plants, and doesn't interfere with blood sugar regulation."

"Chronic sinusitis may also be a factor. Look for that. Is there yeast overgrowth that may be reflecting as increased gas or frequent clearing of the throat? All of these problems can have an effect on mental function, too."

"Then, you should optimize hormones. It's reasonable to try a trial of **Armour Thyroid** in most people with unexplained chronic confusion to see if it helps. A recent study showed that even a low normal thyroid hormone in women was associated with more than a doubled risk of developing dementia!"

"If you've got risk factors for heart disease, the doctor should start with a low dose of Armour and work up slowly."

"In men, if the total testosterone is under 400, I would give a low dose of **bio-identical testosterone cream** to bring the total testosterone level to 600 – 800. Use about 25 to 50 mgs of the cream. It's topical; just put it on the skin."

Search for Depression and Mini-Strokes

"Now let's talk about depression. Apathy, lack of interest, anger – all of these can mimic Alzheimer's. Depression usually has an underlying cause. So make sure that they're not depressed, and if they are, treat it."

"I'd also suggest considering a trial of **1 buffered aspirin** a day. Many people are having mini-strokes, which get misdiagnosed as Alzheimer's. The hallmark of mini-strokes is a step-wise loss of function. A family member may say, 'Gee, last week they took a big drop.' Alzheimer's is more gradual. The aspirin can help prevent these mini-strokes. It often improves function, too."

"If their stomachs are sensitive to aspirin, I'd suggest **willow bark**, 120 mg. It's found in health food stores. But go with the aspirin, if you can."

The Brain-Restoring Supplement that Stops Alzheimer's in its Tracks!

"And they may want to try Rember, a new product that has stopped Alzheimer's in its tracks, in some cases. It's been shown to be much more effective than Aricept."

"Rember is simply old-fashioned **methylene blue**, which is old as dirt. It's also cheap and non-patentable, so it's not out there making billions."

"As a prescription, Rember won't be available for several years. But you can get it from a compounding pharmacist, if ordered by a holistic physician."

Alzheimer's and Senility Are Reversible

"The fact is that Alzheimer's affects almost five million Americans. And with an aging population, drug companies believe there's big money to be made in this area. So there's heavy advertising being done for Aricept, which the research suggests has only minimal benefit."

"As we've been discussing, it's tragic that so many elderly folks get a label of dementia slapped on them and a prescription for Aricept at the first sign of confusion. Most doctors do only a cursory look for other causes, at best."

"In addition to the personal tragedy, the financial costs of this approach are overwhelming. It costs $70,000 to $174,000 to care for someone with Alzheimer's over a lifetime. The global costs for care are $248 billion yearly."

"It's just crazy to not aggressively look for and treat simple reversible problems that can cause or aggravate dementia."

Further Information:

Dr. Jacob Teitelbaum's website:
www.endfatigue.com

Dr. Teitelbaum's website provides information on health conditions from A-Z, as does his free iPhone and Android App "Cures A-Z."

Dr. Teitelbaum offers several supplements for sale on his website.

Chapter 14

Which Fish Oil Works Best?

Fish oil may be the universal supplement. Almost every natural-minded doctor I spoke to recommends it for brain health. In fact, just as I was writing this, a new study popped on my screen:

Rhode Island Hospital study identifies fish oil's impact on cognition and brain structure

PROVIDENCE, R.I. – Researchers at Rhode Island Hospital's Alzheimer's Disease and Memory Disorders Center have found positive associations between fish oil supplements and cognitive functioning as well as differences in brain structure between users and non-users of fish oil supplements. The findings suggest possible benefits of fish oil supplements on brain health and aging. The results were reported at the recent International Conference on Alzheimer's Disease, in Paris, France.

The study was led by Lori Daiello, Pharm.D, a research scientist at the Rhode Island Hospital Alzheimer's Disease and Memory Disorders Center. Data for the analyses was obtained from the Alzheimer's Disease Neuroimaging Initiative (ADNI), a large multi-center, NIH-funded study that followed older adults with normal cognition, mild cognitive impairment, and Alzheimer's Disease for over three years with periodic memory testing and brain MRIs.

Daiello says, "In the imaging analyses for the entire study population, we found a significant positive association between fish oil supplement use and average brain volumes in two critical areas utilized in memory and thinking (cerebral cortex and hippocampus), as well as smaller brain ventricular volumes compared to non-users at any given time in the study. In other words, fish oil use was associated with less brain shrinkage in patients taking these supplements during the ADNI study compared to those who didn't report using them."

Less brain shrinkage is surely a very good thing!

Now it's quite possible that you're already taking fish oil. After all, it's one of the most popular supplements, and its benefits for the heart are widely hailed. But *which* fish oil should you take?

I asked the doctors I interviewed for their views on this raging controversy. Here's some expert advice to help you navigate your way through the fish oil maze.

Vectomega – A Major Breakthrough in Fish Oil and Omega-3 Science

Surprisingly, the best fish oil may not be an oil, at all. Instead, it could be Vectomega, an Omega-3 phospholipid complex derived from salmon heads.

Dr. Jacob Teitelbaum is a big believer in Vectomega, a new product developed in France that draws on some very old folk wisdom.

"Fish heads were considered the best in my old eastern European family," Dr. Teitelbaum told me. "It's an old wives' tale. Well, Vectomega comes from salmon brains, and it turns out grandma was right. She called fish heads 'brain food' for a reason. The brain is made of DHA, the same substance as found in fish oil."

In 2001, the French government asked researchers to investigate potential uses for salmon. This research project gave rise to the "Vectorization" process that produces Vectomega.

Vectomega is farmed from salmon in deep water fjords in Europe, and processed for maximum purity and bioavailability.

In fact, studies show it's *absorbed up to 50 times better than traditional fish oils*!

Pure, Bioidentical and Money-Saving!

Dr. Teitelbaum explained his thoughts on the necessity of fish oil, and why he regards Vectomega as significantly superior to normal fish oils.

"If you suffer from depression, poor memory or a number of other conditions, there's a good chance that you suffer from Omega-3 deficiency and would benefit from adding fish oil to your diet."

"With most of the brain being made of fish oil (as DHA), it's not surprising that consuming fish oil has been shown to reduce existing depression and help with postpartum depression, ADHD, bipolar illness and even schizophrenia. Even in healthy people, supplementing with fish oil decreases anger and anxiety and increases vigor while also improving various types of attention, cognitive and physiological functions — including overall mood."

"Vectomega is so much more effective than normal fish oil that the manufacturer's recommended dose for healthy people is just one tablet per day!"

"Vectomega delivers *bioidentical* EPA (eicosapentaenoic acid) and DHA (docosahexaenoic acid) bound to its natural carrier, called phospholipids, for absorption that is out of this world. A single tablet can have the same effect as 12 standard fish oil gelcaps."

"Here's how they do it:

"Most fish oils are extracted from small, cold-water fish, including sardines, anchovies, herring, and other mixed fish. But then the fish undergo *a lot* of processing. The "cooling and pressing" steps, for example, bring the raw material close to boiling and coagulate the naturally-occurring proteins in the fish. This creates its own problems, as it requires large quantities of solvents (hexane and methanol to name two of them), and the need to reprocess the toxic waste that this method generates."

"But this heat method also alters the *position* of the fatty acids."

"Vectomega uses a gentle, cold water and enzyme process called "vectorization" to extract naturally occurring marine *phospholipids* along with the omega-3 fatty acids DHA and EPA. With vectorization, omega-3 fatty acids are retained in their *natural* position, making them absolutely identical to the omega-3 fatty acids in the human brain. This perfect match allows the body to absorb and use the fatty acids much more efficiently…"

"I've switched all my patients previously on fish oil to the new Vectomega form. It's pure, bioidentical, saves them money and at only 1-2 tablets a day is as effective as 10-12 regular fish oil gelcaps."

Dr. Teitelbaum recommended a number of products to me, which I've written about here, including **Vectomega**, **CuraMed** (curcumin) and the multi-vitamin powder, **Energy Revitalization System**. I asked him if he is affiliated with the manufacturing companies.

He asked me to note, "Though Dr. Teitelbaum serves on the Scientific Advisory Boards of several companies, and helps them design products (including some of the ones mentioned here), he takes no money from any supplement or pharmaceutical companies, with his royalties going to charity."

Krill Oil Versus Vectomega?

I was curious about how Vectomega stacked up against krill oil, which in recent years has become wildly popular. In fact, according to *Nutrition Business Journal*, sales of krill oil are skyrocketing so high that they're outpacing fish oil in percentage of growth.

Health enthusiasts are embracing krill oil because it's a better bet for delivering Omega-3 fatty acids. Krill oil carries its Omega-3s through phospholipids, which are easier to absorb than fish oil's triglycerides.

But it turns out that Vectomega offers the same great deal as krill oil, carrying its Omega-3s in a stream of phospholipids, too. According to its manufacturer, Vectomega is the *first* fish source Omega-3 fatty acid that's delivered by phospholipids. And Vectomega enhances the absorption of Omega-3 fatty acids up to **50-fold** over fish oil!

Here are 3 more advantages of Vectomega over krill oil:

- Vectomega is processed without heat, chemicals or solvents. Its extraction process uses only enzymes and a cold water flush to produce Vectomega from salmon. Krill oil's extraction process can involve heat, chemicals and solvents.

- Unlike both fish and krill oil, Vectomega is not an oil. Therefore, it's chemically stable and not prone to going rancid.

- Krill fishing is now banned off the coasts of California, Oregon and Washington, because of possible environmental concerns. In May, 2010, Whole Foods announced it was withdrawing krill oil from its stores, stating, "Krill are an important source of food for marine animals including penguins, seals, and whales in the Antarctic. Declines of some predator populations in the areas where the krill fishery operates suggest that fishery management needs to better understand how to evaluate the prey requirements of other marine species in order to set sustainable catch levels for krill."

It seems that Vectomega more than holds its own against krill oil.

Microalgae Oil Delivers High DHA

Interestingly, the other fish oil that came highly recommended is also not a fish oil, technically speaking. Dr. Eric Udell of Naturopathic Health Associates in Arizona recommends **microalgae oil** for Alzheimer's patients.

"Microalgae oil is produced by little plankton that little fish eat," explained Dr. Udell. "It's particularly high in DHA and has other health benefits. A study of those taking Aricept and microalgae oil found that those taking both did better."

In fact, the way that fish obtain their Omega-3s is by eating microalgae. When you consume microalgae oil, you eliminate the middleman, so to speak. You're getting your DHA straight from the source, without the dilution of it passing through a fish.

Many people have a big concern about toxins in fish, such as mercury, which could get passed to them through fish oil. When you take microalgae oil, you don't have to worry about consuming the contaminants found in free roaming fish. That's because microalgae oil is extracted from cultured microalgae, so it's free from contaminants.

Of course, you want to get as much DHA as possible from your fish oil. So it's interesting to note that one manufacturer of microalgae oil claims that it provides *250% more DHA per unit than fish oil*!

They also promise another big, health-boosting benefit from microalgae oil. Apparently, it contains the optimum balance of DHA to EPA, the two omega-3 fatty acids found in fish oil.

It's relevant to note that a 2007 study conducted at the University of California, Los Angeles found that supplements of DHA can reduce levels of an enzyme linked to Alzheimer's.

The researchers, who published their work in *The Journal of Neuroscience*, also found that DHA encouraged the production of a protein that fights off brain plaque associated with Alzheimer's. **DHA, they wrote, "may play an important role in preventing LOAD (late-onset Alzheimer's disease)."**

Microalgae oil's high DHA content could make it a highly attractive choice for your Alzheimer's tool kit.

Sources:

Interviews with Dr. Jacob Teitelbaum and Dr. Eric Udell

Dr. Teitelbaum's website
www.endfatigue.com

Vectomega
www.vectomega.com

Vectomega Omega-3 Extract From Salmon Superior to Fish and Krill Oil
April 26, 2011
http://www.europharmausa.com/press-releases/101/april-26-2011-vectomega-omega-3-extract-from-salmon-superior-to-fish-and-krill-oil/

LifeSpan News
"Rhode Island Hospital Study Identifies Fish Oil's Impact on Cognition and Brain Structure"
August 17, 2011
http://www.rhodeislandhospital.org/wtn/Page.asp?PageID=WTN000083

Source-Omega
Benefits of Microalgae Oil
http://www.source-omega.com/omega-3s-are-safe.htm

Nutraingredients.com
"Late-onset Alzheimer's slowed by DHA omega-3"
Stephen Daniells
January 25, 2008
www.nutraingredients.com/Research/Late-onset-Alzheimer-s-slowed-by-DHA-omega-3

Chapter 15

Take Coenzyme Q10 for Dementia; Then Ride a Motorcycle!

Co-Q10 is one of the absolutely essential brain supplements. Almost every doctor I spoke to recommended taking it to combat Alzheimer's.

You may already be taking Co-Q10 for your heart, because its phenomenal cardiovascular effects are quite well-known. But did you realize its brain-boosting abilities may be even more remarkable?

Here's why.

Discover the Spark Plug for Your Brain Cells

Imagine Co-Q10 as a spark plug for your cells. Like a spark plug that starts a car engine, Co-Q10 ignites energy in every cell in your body.

Specifically, it enables the production of adenosine triphosphate (ATP), an essential carrier of cellular energy. Ninety-five percent of your body's energy is generated from ATP! Amazingly, ATP is the main energy source for every organism in the world, from the lowliest bacteria to humans.

When you're young and healthy, Co-Q10 is found in abundance in your brain. After all, your brain is the most metabolically active organ, so it craves a constant supply of Co-Q10 to stay at peak energy.

But, as you grow older, getting enough Co-Q10 may be tricky. Low Co-Q10 levels are all too common in the elderly, dragging down cognitive speed and impairing memory, concentration and clarity.

CoQ10 Protects Your Brain from Free Radical Damage

And Co-Q10 does much more than energize your brain with ATP production; it also acts as a superior antioxidant. Without enough Co-Q10, your brain is at serious risk for damage from free radicals.

These unstable molecules are relentless in sabotaging cellular structure. They target brain cells in the hippocampus, where Alzheimer's starts, causing them to malfunction and die.

But, thankfully, unlike most antioxidants, Co-Q10 can sneak into fatty brain cell membranes, because it's fat-soluble. Inside the membrane, Co-Q10 is perfectly positioned to safeguard brain cells and de-activate free radicals.

And not only can Co-Q10 help to prevent free radical attack, it can also mop up and repair messy cellular damage that free radicals inflict.

Unfortunately, the chances are excellent that right this minute, your brain lacks sufficient Co-Q10 to protect it from free radicals.

Why do I make that educated guess? Two reasons.

Are You Taking Any of These Common Prescription Drugs?

You already know that Co-Q10 helps produce the vital cellular fuel ATP. But what produces Co-Q10?

It turns out that Co-Q10 is manufactured from the amino acid tyrosine, in cahoots with a baker's dozen of vitamins.

And most people on the Standard American Diet (SAD) don't get enough vitamins and minerals to synthesize healthy levels of Co-Q10 for brain protection. Add in the difficulties of many older people with malabsorption of nutrients in their food, and you have a perfect recipe for inadequate Co-Q10.

Now here's the second big reason you may require supplementation of Co-Q10. **Dozens of commonly prescribed medications leech Co-Q10 from your system**!

From cholesterol-lowering medicines like **statins** to **beta blockers** and **antidiabetic prescriptions**, drugs that are taken by millions of people undermine the body's ability to chemically process Co-Q10.

Dr. David Perlmutter, a renowned neurologist in Florida, wrote *The Better Brain Book*, in which he lists common prescription drugs that interfere with Co-Q10 production. By the way, Dr. Perlmutter's book is excellent, and I recommend you read it for in-depth explanations of how to protect your brain from aging.

Take a look at Dr. Perlmutter's list of Co-Q10 inhibitors and see how many of these drugs you're currently taking.

- **Antidepressants**

  Generic Names: Amitriptyline, Desipramine, Doxepin, Imipramine, Nortriptyline, Protriptyline

  Brand Names: Elavil, Norpramin, Sinequan, Tofranil, Aventil, Pamelor, Vivactil

- **Antipsychotic Drugs**

  Generic Name: Haloperidol

  Brand Name: Haldol

- **Blood-Pressure Lowering Drugs**

  Generic Names: Atenolol, Bisoprolol, Clonidine, Hydrochlorothiazide (HCTZ), Nadolol, Metoprolol, Pindolol, Propranolol

  Brand Names: Tenormin, Zebeta, Catapres, Aldactazide, Capozide, Combipres, Dyazide, HydroDIURIL, Hyzaar, Lopressor-HCT, Lotensin HCT, Maxide, Microzide, Moduretic, Prinzide, Vaseretic, Zestoretic, Corgard, Lopressor, Toprol, Visken, Inderal

- **Cholesterol-Lowering Drugs**

  Generic Names: Atorvastatin, Fluvastatin, Lovastatin, Pravastatin, Simvastatin

  Brand Names: Lipitor, Lescol, Mevacor, Pravachol, Zocor

- **Antidiabetic Drugs**

  Generic Names: Glipizide, Glyburide, Tolazamide

  Brand Names: Glucotrol, DiaBeta, Glynase, Micronase, Tolinase

Lancet Study: Alzheimer's Patient Now Rides A Motorcycle!

Co-Q10's unique qualities have long intrigued researchers, who have put its brain-building powers to the test.

I guarantee you'll love this clinical study that was published in the British medical journal, *Lancet*. It followed the remarkable improvements of patients with severe dementia, who were administered a regimen of **Co-Q10, vitamin B6 and iron**.

As long as they took this supplemental combination, their symptoms got better. And in some cases, those improvements were <u>dramatic</u>.

Here's how the researcher describes the outcome for one severe dementia patient: "Her daily activity improved from Stage 5 (moderate Alzheimer's disease) to 1 (normal). She had increased blood flow to the cerebral cortex and decreased symptoms of clinical dementia…*She now rides a motorcycle*."

Take a minute to absorb that mind-boggling news. *A patient with severe dementia improved so much that she now puts on a helmet, hops on a motorbike and speeds down the road with full confidence!*

Co-Q10 surely has some awe-inspiring powers!

Stunning News for Parkinson's Patients: Study Shows 44% Less Decline

In 2002, the Archives of Neurology published the results of a Co-Q10 study funded by the National Institute of Neurological Disorders and Stroke. This investigation was the first placebo-controlled, multicenter clinical trial of Co-Q10. And its implications for battling Parkinson's could be staggering.

Led by the late Clifford Shults, M.D., of the University of California, San Diego (UCSD) School of Medicine, the study looked at 80 Parkinson's patients at 10 centers across the country to determine if Co-Q10 is safe, and if it can slow the rate of functional decline.

The results of this 16-month clinical trial were nothing short of jaw-dropping.

"After an initial screening and baseline blood tests, the patients were randomly divided into four groups. Three of the groups received coenzyme Q_{10} at three different doses (300 mg/day, 600 mg/day, and 1,200 mg/day), along with vitamin E, while a fourth group received a matching placebo that contained vitamin E alone."

"During the study period, the group that received the largest dose of coenzyme Q_{10} (1,200 mg/day) had **44 percent less decline in mental function**, motor (movement) function, and ability to carry out activities of daily living, such as feeding or dressing themselves. The greatest effect was on activities of daily living. The groups that received 300 mg/day and 600 mg/day developed slightly less disability than the placebo group, but the effects were less than those in the group that received the highest dosage of coenzyme Q_{10}."

"The groups that received coenzyme Q_{10} also had significant increases in the level of coenzyme Q_{10} in their blood and a significant increase in energy-producing reactions within their mitochondria."

44% less decline in mental function…That's breathtaking news!

How Much Co-Q10 Should You Take?

If you're taking prescription medicines that deplete your stock of Co-Q10, you may need to take additional supplementation.

Dr. David Perlmutter recommends that people who are experiencing significant loss of cognitive function or who are at high risk of mental decline take 200 milligrams of Co-Q10.

He also advises that if you're taking prescription drugs that reduce Co-Q10 levels, you should take an additional 100 milligrams, for a total daily dose of 300 milligrams. Dr. Perlmutter suggests that you take 200 milligrams in the morning and 100 milligrams in the evening, for maximum benefit.

On the other hand, Dr. Jeffrey Morrison of the Morrison Health Center in New York City recommends a much higher dose for Alzheimer's patients. He suggests to his Alzheimer's patients that they take 400 mg of Co-Q10 twice a day.

Whatever your daily dosage, you'll want to take enough Co-Q10 to get the full benefits of this uniquely potent brain booster.

What's the best, most bio-available form of Co-Q10?

Not all Co-Q10 is created equal, and you may want to select a form that's far more potent than the standard brands.

According to *Cancer Defeated* Publications, "95 percent of the Co-Q10 in your blood is in a form called *ubiquinol*. But the form of Co-Q10 found in nearly all supplements is *ubiquinone*. Your body has to convert the ubiquinone in the capsules into ubiquinol, and it's not very efficient about doing that."

"The reason supplement makers market the "inferior" form is that it doesn't spoil as easily. The more potent form — ubiquinol — is very reactive with oxygen and oxidizes when exposed to air. In fact, the form found in the pills — ubiquinone — IS the oxidized form of Co-Q10. You could say the Co-Q10 in pills is the "spoiled" form!"

"But I've got good news: researchers have found a way to stabilize ubiquinol so it doesn't oxidize, and you can now obtain this superior form of Co-Q10 in supplements. Animal studies and some individual case studies in humans have confirmed that the superior form really is more effective."

Dr. Robert Rowen, who has created a formula that contains ubiquinol, says that ubiquinol is absorbed **8 times more efficiently** than the standard form of Co-Q10.

According to Dr. Rowen, "That means just 25 mg per day of ubiquinol provides virtually the same high Co-Q10 blood levels as 200 mg of standard Co-Q10."

Ubiquinol costs more than the standard Co-Q10 supplements. However, you may discover it works out to be a cost-effective choice, since you'll probably need to take smaller doses to get the same brain-nourishing benefits.

Sources:

The Better Brain Book
David Perlmutter, M.D., FACN and Carol Colman
Riverhead Books, 2004

Cancer Defeated
"The Powerful Cancer Cure Locked Inside Your Cells"
By Lee Euler
Issue 21
http://cancerdefeatedpublications.com/newsletters/The-Powerful-Cancer-Cure-Locked-Inside-Your-Cells.html

National Institute of Neurological Disorders and Strokes
Study Suggests Coenzyme Q10 Slows Functional Decline in Parkinson's Disease

Monday, October 14, 2002
http://www.ninds.nih.gov/news_and_events/news_articles/pressrelease_parkinsons_coenzymeq10_101402.htm

Chapter 16

Meet the Naturopathic Healers: "We Can Prolong Quality of Life For A Long, Long Time"

Is it possible to help reverse Alzheimer's with a few drops of a highly diluted natural substance? According to some dedicated naturopathic physicians whom I interviewed, the answer is, "Absolutely."

Naturopathic physicians favor a holistic approach that encourages the body's innate capacity to heal. They try to employ the least invasive measures possible, and to avoid unnecessary surgery and drugs.

The naturopathic physicians whom I interviewed all use homeopathic medicine as part of their tool kit. Homeopathy was developed more than two hundred years ago by a German physician named Samuel Hahnemann. He formulated the principle of "like cures like," which states that a disease can be cured by a substance that produces similar symptoms in healthy people.

Homeopathy uses very small doses of highly diluted natural substances to stimulate the body's own healing powers. In fact, its principle of dilutions (or "law of minimum dose") states that the *lower* the dose of the medication, the *greater* its effectiveness. Homeopaths create an individualized treatment for each patient, based on extensive inquiry into their health history and symptoms.

So can homeopathy improve the lives of Alzheimer's patients? Listen to these exciting and hopeful stories from three distinguished naturopathic physicians, who have witnessed the power of homeopathic remedies.

All three doctors embrace a philosophy of taking time with patients to understand their complete medical situation. They carefully probe for their patients' nutritional deficits and underlying infections, as well as any hormonal imbalances. And then, they deftly use homeopathy to help bring the body back into balance.

How Dr. Eric Udell Approaches Alzheimer's

Dr. Eric Udell graduated from the Southwest College of Naturopathic Medicine. Following his residency training, he completed a two-year post-doctoral fellowship in Homeopathy, *the first fellowship of its kind in the United States.*

Now an Assistant Professor of Homeopathy at SCNM, Dr. Udell often tackles challenging cases and serious or chronic illness. Helping his patients recover using natural, safe, non-toxic remedies gives Dr. Udell deep satisfaction and has given him special expertise in treating autoimmune diseases including rheumatoid arthritis and lupus.

I asked Dr. Udell to tell me about his approach to Alzheimer's. "The old adage that an ounce of prevention is worth a pound of cure is more true of Alzheimer's than of almost any other disease. So, first, we should ask what can we do to decrease our chances of getting it," Dr. Udell said.

"Next, if we don't have any therapies right now that can grow new brain cells, then what can we do to prevent further damage to the still-functioning brain cells. If we detect Alzheimer's early, we can prolong quality of life and independent living for a long, long time."

"I currently have a gentleman who's 89 years old, who was diagnosed with Alzheimer's in 2001. For the last ten years, he's been living independently. In fact, he was driving until the last six months. We managed to stop the progression for a very extended period of time."

"He's been taking homeopathy – classical homeopathy that's individualized. If a patient comes in with any kind of dementia, there are probably a couple of hundred potential homeopathic medicines. We need to figure out what's best for the person, which we do by finding out his exact symptoms and how they manifest."

"Let's say the symptom is confusion. The exact nature and flavor of confusion varies. One person has trouble recognizing people and names. Another person does fine with that, but can't remember where they put anything down, such as their keys or glasses. Another person is delusional. He thinks people are breaking into his house and stealing things."

"From a diagnostic standpoint, those manifestations all lead to a different homeopathic treatment. We look to the whole person and their symptoms, including their emotions. Some are more prone to anxiety or depression or irritability."

"For instance, this gentleman when I first started working with him had painful leg cramps. He also had vertigo and choked on his food. These symptoms helped me figure out the particulars of his homeopathic treatment."

"When we're able to do a good job, it works by stimulating an innate healing response. It reinstates a higher level of function, so symptoms begin to improve without side effects."

"This gentleman stopped having vertigo and leg cramps and no longer choked on his food. And there was no further progression of confusion and cognitive issues."

"In addition, I put him on supplements of **acetyl carnitine.** He was already on **Aricept,** and patients who take Aricept plus acetyl carnitine do better."

"And we put him on **microalgae oil**. This oil is produced by little plankton that the little fish eat. It's particularly high in DHA and has other health benefits. A study of those taking Aricept and microalgae oil found that those taking both did better."

"And I also put him on **MCT oil**, which is derived from coconut oil. MCT oil is an alternative fuel for the brain, instead of glucose. It's safe. There's little chance of it harming anyone."

"I'd make these three components – acetyl carnitine, microalgae oil and MCT oil – part of a standard Alzheimer's supplement regimen. They're all very safe and non-toxic."

As Dr. Udell told me the story of his patient, I found myself marveling with admiration. An 89-year-old man, living independently and driving, *ten years* after an Alzheimer's diagnosis! Now that's encouraging!

And here's what Dr. Udell's colleague at Arizona Natural Health Center had to say…

Meet Dr. Tara Peyman of Arizona Natural Health Center

I was excited to talk to Dr. Tara Peyman, because she's one of the few naturopathic doctors who specializes in mental disorders. Her primary passion is the homeopathic and integrative treatment of bipolar disorder and mental illness.

Dr. Peyman was trained by some of the best classical homeopathic physicians in the United States and internationally. Her practice focuses on addressing the underlying causes of illness, and empowering the patient to treat those deeper concerns using homeopathy and natural medicine.

Dr. Peyman treats people suffering from depression, anxiety, schizophrenia, OCD, PTSD, and many other conditions. She can assist patients in either tapering off psychiatric medications, or integrating them with naturopathic care, if necessary.

"It's important for the public to know that Alzheimer's is reversible in most cases, especially if it's treated early," Dr. Peyman told me. "We can help people be more functional and productive, and happier in their lives."

"The first thing I do is to ask the patient to tell the story of what they've seen and noticed. And then a family member tells me what they've noticed, so we can put together the story. I'm trying to get a real clear medical history and timeline of symptoms. For instance, was it a sudden onset? In that case, it's something different than Alzheimer's, which is typically slow and insidious."

"I like to run blood tests and look for other problems, such as thyroid problems. They're common in mental decline, and can contribute to depression or other mood problems. And they also can cause confusion, brain fog and memory lapses. Thyroid problems become more common as we age, especially in women, but even in men over 65. They're not looked for enough."

"There is so much overlap between hypothyroidism and the initial presentation of Alzheimer's. If they do have a serious thyroid problem, I'd put them on a natural thyroid medication like Armour. It's the same as synthetic medicine, but has less additives."

"I'd also look for hormonal and chemical imbalances underneath. Blood sugar imbalance can contribute to cognitive and memory problems. Vitamin D levels are typically low in the elderly. Iron and B12 deficiencies can also contribute, but not as much as the thyroid."

"For instance, I treated a patient who no longer needs any help. She came in with memory problems. She couldn't focus or concentrate. She had no motivation and cried all the time. She felt defeated."

"Now since she was in her 60s and had memory problems, somebody might think it's early Alzheimer's. But she had a struggling thyroid and her blood sugar was uncontrolled. I put her on a healthy low glycemic diet with lots of veggies and whole foods. And I put her on homeopathic treatment."

"She improved dramatically with just the dietary changes and homeopathic remedies. Her cholesterol and blood sugar normalized. Her thyroid improved dramatically. Her mood went up and her knee pain went away. She no longer had the cognitive issues."

"Homeopathic medicines work on a deeper level to stop the damage from happening in the first place. They improve the quality of a person's health as a dynamic whole, helping on a cellular level."

"You can see patients improve on lots of different levels. I had a patient come in with mild Alzheimer's, Stage 3. She was having problems with memory and cognition."

"I gave her a homeopathic remedy and started just with that. Lachesis is the name of the homeopathic medicine I used. It's one of the good ones commonly used for Alzheimer's."

"Well, this patient also had chronic migraines and stuttering and a history of depression. After I gave her the lachesis, she dramatically improved. Her daughter was amazed right away at how much happier she was."

"Her memory and focus came back. She felt upbeat and started being productive around the house. Her headaches went away and her stammering got better. So it worked on many levels."

"One of the nice things about homeopathic remedies is that they don't interfere with conventional medicines such as high blood pressure medicines. In fact, homeopathy might reduce the need for them, so patients should make sure to get monitored to see if they can reduce their medication."

"Homeopathy is unique. It's individualized to each person. And the thing that's most exciting to me is that I've seen the biggest improvements of health come from homeopathic treatment."

Meet Dr. Farhang Khosh of Natural Medical Care in Kansas

Dr. Farhang Khosh, N.D., and his brother, Dr. Mehdi Khosh, N.D., run Natural Medical Care, with two offices in Kansas. The Khosh brothers formerly worked at the Kansas Clinic of Traditional Medicine and Via Christi Integrative Center in Wichita, Kansas. Both brothers have published numerous papers on naturopathic approaches to disease.

The Khosh brothers accomplish health care using clinical nutrition, botanical medicine, homeopathic medicine and physical medicine, including acupuncture and lifestyle counseling.

Dr. Farhang Khosh received his Doctorate of Naturopathic Medicine from Bastyr University, a nationally accredited naturopathic medical school in Seattle. He graduated from the University of Kansas where he earned his bachelor's degree in Biochemistry and did advanced work in Molecular Biology.

I asked Dr. Khosh how he diagnoses a patient with Alzheimer's.

"I often look for clues from their reaction to a blood test," he replied. "Let's say a daughter and mother bring in the father, because they suspect Alzheimer's. Usually, they come in the afternoon, around two or three o'clock. I talk to the patient, and he understands what's going on and can engage in conversation."

"I say, let's do a blood test and check your lipids, blood sugar, thyroid and B12 levels. Come back tomorrow, and make sure to fast before the test."

"Now here's the hallmark of what may be going on. When they bring him in the next day and he's been fasting, he's completely confused. He doesn't know who I am or why he's there. So it could be that his blood sugar is so low, his brain isn't focusing."

"I had one patient like this. His blood sugar tested so low, it was 42. The normal fasting range is 65 – 99. His brain was not getting enough glucose to function."

"It could be Alzheimer's, that's getting worse with low blood sugar. Or it could be that it's not Alzheimer's; he's confused because of his low blood sugar."

"I decided to just optimize his blood sugar and see what happens. I put him on an eight week eating program, and taught him how to eat small, but more frequent meals, heavy on protein. He was eating simple carbs, not complex carbs and protein."

"I also gave him **chromium picolinate** which balances blood sugar. I started with 200 micrograms, and increased it to 200 micrograms twice a day, with breakfast and lunch."

"Well, there's been a huge difference in coherence. He started feeling much better, and we test him every three weeks to make sure his blood sugar is stabilizing."

"It turned out he does have Alzheimer's, and still has some short term memory loss. But the beauty of this is he functions so well, we forget that he has Alzheimer's."

"Now another common issue is urinary tract infections. A majority of older people gets them, and when it becomes really bad, kidney function isn't optimal. When the kidney doesn't function well, toxin levels go way up in the blood and can interfere with brain function."

"A person can become confused, so we need to find and take care of the infection. We also need to increase the oxygen in the brain. I may have the patient do deep breathing, and get oxygen supplied from a mask, so they can breathe efficiently."

"I treated an 84-year-old male who was a very powerful business executive. He was perfectly fine until he had sepsis from a urinary tract infection. He went to the Mayo Clinic, where they gave him massive antibiotics. Then they sent him home and told him he had Alzheimer's."

"In just four weeks, you had a high level executive go from that kind of functioning to where he couldn't remember his name."

"I put him on a high dose of **Co-Enzyme Q10**, 1200 mgs a day. I also gave him **glutathione** which is one of the most powerful antioxidants, 300 mg in a 3 ml solution to be nebulized."

"I had him for two months while he lived with family here. After the third week, there was nothing wrong with him. He engaged in long conversations with me, and was giving me tips on how to make money."

"He had been so depressed, because since his Alzheimer's diagnosis, the family wasn't comfortable with him making decisions. He had always been the decision maker. Well, after eight weeks, he was back to making the majority of the decisions in the family."

"He was also depressed because he liked to drive his wife around in the golf cart, and with the Alzheimer's diagnosis, he couldn't do that. Now he's back to driving his wife around in the golf cart and enjoying himself."

"My philosophy is even if a patient does have Alzheimer's, you can alleviate symptoms by checking their blood sugar and oxygenation. And make sure they take supplements like **gingko** that increase blood flow to the brain, and **turmeric (curcumin)** as an anti-inflammatory agent.

Finding A Homeopathic Physician

I asked Dr. Eric Udell how to go about finding a good homeopathic doctor. He suggested utilizing the website of The National Center for Homeopathy, which can be found at www. homeopathic.org.

Dr. Udell also noted that homeopathy is practiced by some naturopathic physicians. The American Association of Naturopathic Physicians has a searchable database at www.naturopathic. org

Dr. Tara Peyman cautioned that not all naturopathic doctors are extensively trained in homeopathic medicine. She said there are lots of people who say they practice homeopathy, but don't do it in the best way. They may use different methods which stray from the original techniques with which homeopathy is supposed to be practiced.

Dr. Peyman suggested that you make sure your doctor is licensed as a naturopathic physician, and went to an accredited four-year medical school.

"There are only four schools like that in the country," Dr. Peyman told me. "I went to Southwest College of Naturopathic Medicine. We have Dr. Stephen Messer who practices it, as it was originally meant to be practiced."

"The other four-year accredited medical schools are Bastyr University in Seattle; National College of Natural Medicine in Portland, Oregon; and the University of Bridgeport College of Naturopathic Medicine in Bridgeport, Connecticut."

"You can search online. Each school has a website and an alumni page."

"Also, we have six doctors practicing here at Arizona Natural Health Center. We all do free 15-minute telephone consultations, so we may be able to help."

Further Information:

Dr. Eric Udell

Dr. Tara Peyman

Arizona Natural Health Center
1250 E. Baseline Road, Suite 104, Tempe, Arizona 85283
Phone: (480) 456-0402 | Fax: (480) 456-0409
www.aznaturalhealth.com

Dr. Farhang Khosh
Natural Medical Care
4935 Research Parkway
Lawrence, KS 66047
(785) 749-2255
www.naturalmedicalcare.com

Chapter 17

Which Vital Vitamins Does Your Brain Lack?

A good place to begin talking about vitamins is by looking at what's on your plate. Is your diet SAD? In other words, do you follow the Standard American Diet (SAD), which is heavy on processed foods, sugar, simple carbs, and saturated fats?

Well, if you do, you're starving your brain of the nutrients it's begging for. Upgrading what you eat can make a huge difference in your overall vitality and mental clarity.

Nita Scoggan, whom you met in Chapter 9, dove into researching brain-healthy food when her beloved husband Bill developed Alzheimer's. And what she found shocked her.

"Potatoes, white bread, corn…All of Bill's favorite foods that he grew up with were making his brain sluggish!" she exclaimed.

One study that was reported in the *American Journal of Clinical Nutrition* showed that fewer than 5% of the study participants consumed the recommended daily amounts (RDAs) of all their needed vitamins and minerals. What's really frightening is that this study was conducted in Beltsville, Maryland, on U.S. Department of Agriculture (USDA) research center employees!

Every single vitamin and nutritional mineral is important in some way to your wellbeing. You don't want to miss out on any, because you'll pay for the shortage in the worst possible way - with your health.

So which foods adequately nourish your brain?

You've already heard from some of the doctors I interviewed: eat plenty of **vegetables, fruits, complex carbohydrates, lean protein, healthy fats, seeds and nuts**.

But let's examine the do's and don'ts of brain-healthy eating a bit more closely.

Among other sources, I drew on advice from Dr. David Perlmutter in *The Better Brain Book,* Dr. Vincent Fortanasce in *The Anti-Alzheimer's Prescription* and Jack Challem in *The Inflammation Syndrome* for this list.

Brain-Boosting Foods:

• **Vegetables** (five to six servings a day): leafy greens; cruciferous veggies like broccoli, watercress, kale, cabbage, brussel sprouts, cauliflowers, Swiss chard; onions, avocado, bell peppers, celery, carrots, fennel, string beans, scallions, etc.

• **Fish** (two to three servings a week): herring, mackerel, halibut, sardines, Alaskan sockeye salmon, bass, cod, trout, lobster, snapper, sole, etc.

• **Fruit** (two servings a day): apples, apricots, berries, citrus fruits, grapes, kiwi, melons, peaches, plums, pears, etc. Too much fruit can send your blood sugar spiking, so try to stick to two daily servings.

• **Meat**: chicken, turkey, Cornish game hen, buffalo, lean grass-fed beef, lamb, pork, etc.

• You can eat chicken, turkey, Cornish game hen and buffalo every day. Twice a week, you can have a meal with beef, lamb or pork.

• **Seeds, Nuts, and Nut Butters** (one serving of nuts and one serving of seeds daily): walnuts, almonds, cashews, peanuts, hazelnuts, pistachios, filberts; pumpkin seeds, sunflower seeds, flax seeds

• **Eggs and Dairy**: Omega 3-enriched eggs; low-fat/non-fat cheeses and yogurt. You can eat up to six to eight eggs a week, and enjoy up to two daily servings of dairy.

• **Protein Powder**: two tablespoons of whey protein

• **Grains and Breads** (one to two daily servings): whole grains, sprouted grains, steel cut oatmeal, buckwheat, barley, quinoa, basmati brown rice, semolina, millet
Note: Whole grain products contain the word *whole*, not *enriched*.

• **Legumes** (one to two daily servings): lentils, beans, chickpeas, lima beans, pink beans, navy beans, cranberry beans, red beans, black beans, white beans, pinto beans, great northern beans, kidney beans

• **Herbs and Spices**: garlic, curcumin, cinnamon, basil, oregano, rosemary, tarragon, etc. Go easy on the salt.

• **Oils**: Olive oil, macadamia nut oil, avocado oil, coconut oil

Brain-Bashing Foods

- **White, Processed Flour**: white bread, rolls, muffins, sweetened cereal, crackers, pasta

- **Highly Processed Foods**: Foods with lots of ingredients, including some you can't identify.

- **Fried Foods**

- **Fatty cuts of meat**, including bacon, brisket, spareribs and deli meats

- **Sugar and sweets**: cookies, candy, cakes, ice cream, frozen yogurt, sorbet, fruit-flavored yogurt, dried fruit, sweetened cereals, soda pop, sweetened tea, fruit juice

- **Sugar Substitutes**: corn syrup, high-fructose corn syrup, brown sugar, concentrated fruit juice, dextrose, fructose, honey, sucrose, powered sugar, maple syrup, molasses

- **Snacks**: chips, pretzels, popcorn, energy bars

- **Hydrogenated oils**: corn oil, margarines with trans-fatty acids, soy oil, squeezable butter, peanut oil, safflower oil, sunflower oil, canola oil, cottonseed oil

- **Foods high in sodium, salt and MSG**

Foods to Limit:

- **Starchy Veggies (limit to no more than one serving a day)**: corn, potatoes, yams, turnips

Why Even the Healthiest Eater May Still Need to Take Vitamins

Now let's assume you're following all these recommendations to the letter. You're eating fresh, healthy, delicious food.

Chances are excellent that you'll still need to take supplemental vitamins, especially if you're battling Alzheimer's.

Here are 3 good reasons why.

- **One**: Older people frequently have problems with malabsorption. As the name suggests, this simply means poor absorption. In other words, even if they eat healthy foods, their bodies are no longer adept at extracting the nutrients from them.

- **Two**: Alzheimer's is a disease of atrophy, in which patients lose appetite and waste away.

They may not be able to eat much; certainly not enough to nourish their bodies with the healing bonanza of nutrients they need.

- **Three**: Many common medications disrupt the proper absorption of nutrients, making the problems discussed above even more severe.

So which supplemental vitamins do Alzheimer's patients need, in what quantity? And what's the best way to supply them?

The Easiest, No Fuss Way to Get Every Nutrient You Need

Dr. Jacob Teitelbaum told me that he's a big believer in keeping things simple. He doesn't like to see Alzheimer's patients gobbling piles of pills all day, so he advises taking a good multivitamin supplement that lays down a solid base of daily nutrition.

He recommends a powdered formula that he helped to create. It's called the **Energy Revitalization System**, and it's available on his website (www.endfatigue.com). Every morning, you take a scoop and mix it with water, a beverage, smoothie or yogurt.

Dr. Teitelbaum explains that the ease and convenience of this nutrient-packed formula offers plenty of advantages:

- Delivers the benefits of over 50 vitamins, minerals and other nutrients for sustained energy

- Replaces the equivalent of 25-35 tablets a day.

- Features malic acid to stimulate the complete burning of fuel for energy and support healthy connective tissue and muscle functioning

- Includes vitamin D3 for immune system and bone support

- Contains amino acids essential to metabolism, immunity and overall health

- Also delivers key nutrients including choline for mental alertness and antioxidants for protection from oxidative stress and free-radical damage

Occasionally, people experience loose stools from a powder. If you do, Dr. Teitelbaum suggests you can take a tablet multi-vitamin, instead. He recommends a brand called **My Favorite Multiple**.

But please heed these two caveats:

1. If you're taking **Coumadin or any other blood-thinner**, don't take these multi-vitamins or ANY supplement without your physician's approval. For other medications, the interactions are generally not significant.

2. Even with a good multi-vitamin, you may need to boost your **Vitamin B12** levels with a series of injections. I'll explain the miraculous powers of B12 in just a minute.

Whether you choose to take a single multi-vitamin, or supplement your diet with separate vitamins, as some doctors recommend, it's a good idea to understand each nutrient's brain-boosting role.

So let's B-gin with B!

B Healthy, Supplement Your B Vitamins

In September 2010, the *Daily Mail*, a British newspaper, splashed a stunning headline across its pages: **10p pill to beat Alzheimer's disease: Vitamin B halts memory loss in breakthrough British trial**. (10p equals 10 pence in England, which is worth about 16 cents in the United States.)

"A simple vitamin pill could prevent millions from suffering the agony of Alzheimer's," the article explained. "**The tablet, costing as little as 10p a day and made up of three vitamin B supplements, cut brain shrinkage linked to memory loss by up to 500 percent.**"

The article described how researchers from Oxford University had conducted a landmark study on 270 pensioners suffering from memory loss that leads to Alzheimer's.

For two years, one group took a tablet containing extremely high doses of vitamins B6, 9 and 12. The other group took a placebo.

After two years, their brains were scanned to evaluate brain shrinkage --- and the group taking the B vitamin tablet had 30 percent less shrinkage, on average.

But, for pensioners with the most serious problems, the results were even better: the vitamin B tablet "halved the shrinkage, and in one extreme case, it cut it five-fold," according to the *Daily Mail*.

The B vitamin group also scored better on memory tests, such as remembering lists.

Professor Helga Refsum, one of the researchers said, "Here we have a very simple solution: you give some vitamins and you seem to protect the brain."

Noted the *Daily Mail*, "The results suggest that a basic cocktail of vitamins can achieve results that have evaded pharmaceutical companies, despite billions of pounds being spent on experimental dementia drugs."

So what makes B vitamins so effective?

B Vitamins Protect the Brain from Deadly Homocysteine

"The single most exciting discovery in Alzheimer's prevention is that the amino acid homocysteine is involved in the development in the disease," wrote Patrick Holford, director of London's Brain Bio Centre, in his book, *The Alzheimer's Prevention Plan.*

Holford regards this insight as key, because homocysteine "is a highly reversible risk factor, involving no recourse to expensive drugs or procedures – just simple dietary changes and B vitamin supplementation."

Why haven't you heard more about homocysteine? 7,000 studies have been published in professional journals about it, and yet, to most doctors, it remains almost completely obscure.

Holford takes a jaundiced view of why the medical community hasn't rushed to embrace this discovery: *there's not enough money in it.*

"The sad truth is that, with no patentable or profitable treatment involved in lowering homocysteine levels, scientists are finding it hard to get their studies funded," he wrote.

Holford speculated that the discovery linking homocysteine to Alzheimer's could ultimately threaten billions of dollars in profits from prescription drugs like Aricept. And companies threatened by such staggering profit loss will aggressively act to protect their turf.

By now, you must be curious about what homocysteine is and what it does that's so important.

Homocysteine is an amino acid produced in the body that should always be kept at low levels. Excess homocysteine circulating in the blood damages the brain in multiple ways. It incites inflammation, kills off cells, and blocks blood delivery to the brain.

Not only that, it boosts the risk of over 50 diseases from heart attacks to strokes and cancer.

And guess which nutrients control homocysteine levels? B vitamins!

If your B vitamin levels are low, in all likelihood, your homocysteine levels are too high. And that imbalance spells danger for your brain.

In 1998, a research team at Oxford University, working with OPTIMA (Oxford Project to Investigate Memory and Ageing) first discovered that Alzheimer's patients exhibited high levels of homocysteine in the blood.

Many studies have since confirmed that finding. Here's a particularly interesting correlation. Alzheimer's is characterized by shrinking of the hippocampus section of the brain; researchers have discovered that homocysteine levels affect the size of the hippocampus.

On a practical note, high homocysteine levels can degrade your mental speed and reaction time, along with your sense of balance. Your hand-eye coordination can suffer, and that means you'll have trouble driving. Say goodbye to your golf and tennis game, too, and many other activities you enjoy.

The ugly fact is that out-of-control homocysteine induces poor concentration and judgment, loss of memory, depression, and physical deterioration.

So what can you do to stomp down those homocysteine levels? Get enough B vitamins!

And that probably means taking B vitamin supplements. It's true that B vitamins abound in meat, fish and eggs. But B vitamins have an unfortunate habit of collapsing when they're microwaved, cooked with high heat, or plunged into cooking fluid.

So, even when you eat B-rich foods, you might not reap their benefits.

And if you're a vegetarian or vegan, you're *really* at risk of low B vitamin levels, especially B12. The best B-vitamin sources are animal products, which you're not eating.

And now it's time to open your medicine cabinet, and check out another reason you may have a B-vitamin deficit.

Do You Take These Common B-Destroying Medicines?

Lots of common prescription drugs interfere with the metabolism of B vitamins. Do you take any of them?

Here are some categories of B-depleting medications:

aspirin; antibiotics for chronic urinary tract infections; antacid and stomach acid suppressors; antidiabetic drugs; asthma drugs; blood pressure-lowering drugs; anticonvulsant drugs; cholesterol-lowering drugs; estrogens; estrogen substitutes; anti-Parkinson's drugs; nonsteroidal anti-inflammatory drugs (NSAIDS); corticosteroids anti-inflammatory drugs.

If you're on these medications, you should be taking daily B vitamin supplementation. And you should **ask your doctor to regularly check your homocysteine levels.**

By the way, did your doctor ever tell you that taking any of these drugs is probably compromising your vitamin B levels and boosting your homocysteine?

Just to drive home what's at stake, consider this recent study of people who had taken part in the Scottish Mental Surveys of 1932 and 1947, which measured childhood intelligence.

When researchers in Scotland tested these older adults for mental sharpness, the best performers had the highest levels of B vitamins and lowest levels of homocysteine!

Now let's put each B vitamin in the spotlight, beginning with the greatest miracle worker of all.

Switch on Your Light with Vitamin B12

Stories abound of Alzheimer's patients coming to life after getting B12 injections. Dr. Ronald Hoffman told me, "If a patient hasn't been properly diagnosed with Vitamin B12 deficiency, we can really light somebody up with a series of injections. They perk right up," said Dr. Hoffman.

How do you know if you're low on B12? Telltale symptoms can include brain fog, dementia, loss of balance, and numbness or tingling in the limbs.

"If you have B12 deficiencies, your energy and concentration are going to be sapped," said Dr. Hoffman.

Some studies show that between 17 to 20 percent of elderly people have vitamin B12 deficiencies.

Every doctor I spoke to emphasized the need to insure adequate B12 levels. And that's a story unto itself, because it so happens that what conventional medical wisdom regards as enough B12 may not be enough, at all.

Dr. Jacob Teitelbaum wrote, "Technically, the B12 level is normal if it is over 208 picograms per deciliter (pg/dL) of blood. However, studies have shown that people can suffer severe and sometimes long-term nerve and brain damage from B12 deficiency even if their levels are as high as 300 pg/dL. Why are the "normal" levels set so low? In part, the normal values were initially set according to what prevents anemia. But the brain's and nervous system's needs for vitamin B12 are often much higher than those of the bone marrow."

As Dr. Teitelbaum points out, B12 is vital for healthy nerves. In fact, one of its most important functions is to protect brain nerve cells from the deterioration of the aging process.

A new study, published in the journal *Neurology*, detailed the results of a B12 clinical trial conducted at Rush University Medical Center in Chicago. Researchers looked at markers of B12 deficiency, including homocysteine levels, in 121 older adults. The subjects took tests measuring their cognitive function. Then, four years later, their total brain volume was measured with an MRI.

"We showed that four out of five markers of B12 deficiency were strongly associated with poor cognitive performance overall, and more specifically, poor episodic memory and perceptual speed," said Christine Tangney, Ph.D., the study's lead author.

And, strikingly, the size of the brain was affected, too. Dr. Tangney's team discovered that adults with high levels of markers for B12 deficiency had significantly smaller brain volume.

And who wants their brain to shrink?

If you're over 60, be aware that people in that age group may develop a condition called atrophic gastritis, which induces B12 deficiency. It mimics the symptoms of indigestion, so it's often overlooked. And to make matters far worse, if you have atrophic gastritis, you could be popping antacids all day, which are B12 destroyers, too.

To increase your body's supply of B12, you can take oral supplements. The recommended dosage is 500 – 1,000 mcg. The most commonly recommended B12 supplements are sublingual; i.e. they're dissolved under the tongue.

However, your doctor may decide you should begin your B12 supplementation with a series of injections that allow for better absorption. Dr. Ronald Hoffman includes a case study on his website in which he gave an Alzheimer's patient a series of B12 shots 3 times weekly for two weeks, then started her on monthly injections.

Whether you take supplements or injections, B12 is so crucial for your brain health that you should put it at the top of your list to discuss with your doctor.

Folic Acid (Vitamin B9) Stimulates Your Brain to Act 9 Years Younger!

"Folic acid is a biggie," Dr. Jacob Teitelbaum told me. "In terms of prevention, folate is one of the most important supplements for memory."

Whether you call it folate, folic acid or vitamin B9, numerous studies document this powerhouse nutrient's special talent for warding off depression, brain fog, apathy, confusion, and memory loss.

Now hold on to your hat, because you're about to read the results of a 3-year study that measured folic acid's effect on cognitive function…and they are simply mind-boggling!

The study, published in the journal *The Lancet*, was a randomized, double blind, controlled trial. It documented the impact of taking 800 micrograms of folic acid on global cognitive function over a 3-year period.

A group of older adults started this FACIT (Folic Acid and Carotid Intima-media Thickness) trial by taking a host of tests for cognition, memory, sensorimotor speed, complex speed, information-processing speed, and word fluency. At the beginning of the trial, the folic acid group and the placebo group scored about the same.

But, after three years of taking 800 micrograms of folic acid every day, the folic acid group had grown sharper, quicker, smarter and just plain younger!

Is memory loss an issue for you? Then here's a fact you may want to memorize: On the test that measured delayed memory recall (how subjects remembered a fifteen-word learning test), **the group taking folic acid had shaved 6 to 9 years off their performance**!

The folic acid group also scored:

• **4.7 years younger for memory**

• **2.1 years younger for information-processing speed**

• **1.7 years younger for sensorimotor speed**

• **1.5 years younger for global cognitive function**

If we examine their blood test results, we'll discover what's turning back the clock in their brains. The folic acid group had increased their folate concentrations by *576 percent*!

And their levels of homocysteine had shrunk by *26 percent*! Since homocysteine is a nasty amino acid that shrinks the hippocampus, murders brain cells and stifles blood delivery to the brain, it's fabulous news that folic acid can so dramatically lower its presence.

And, having low levels of folic acid is specifically associated with Alzheimer's. The results of a long-term study published in *Alzheimer's & Dementia: The Journal of the Alzheimer's Association*, indicate that consuming adequate levels of folic acid is associated with the greatest protection against Alzheimer's disease of <u>any</u> nutrient examined.

Assistant professor of neurology Maria Corrada-Bravo of the University of California Irvine's Institute for Brain Aging and Dementia examined data from the Baltimore Longitudinal Study of Aging, which was begun in 1958 and includes over 1,400 participants.

Dr. Corrada-Bravo noted, "The participants who had intakes at or above the 400 microgram recommended dietary allowance of folate had a 55% reduction in the risk of developing Alzheimer's. But most people who reached that level did so by taking folic acid supplements, which suggests that many people do not get the recommended amounts of folate in their diets."

If you're battling Alzheimer's, a recommended dosage is 800 mcg daily.

Thiamine (Vitamin B1) Improves Mood, Energy, Clarity

Thiamine, also known as vitamin B1, is crucial for brain metabolic functions. It plays a big part in heart function, too, contributing to numerous enzyme processes, and the regulation of nerve and muscle cells.

Thiamine isn't stored well in the body, so you can quickly grow depleted of it – especially, if you're an alcoholic. Unfortunately, heavy drinkers can develop a thiamine-caused disorder called Wernicke's encephalopathy, characterized by confusion, vision problems, and lack of balance.

Thiamine is used therapeutically in dementia, anxiety, neuropathy, fatigue, alcoholism, confusion, depression, pain, memory loss, and disequilibrium.

In a double blind study by Dr. David Benton, supplementation with vitamin B1 improved mood—possibly by increasing synthesis of acetylcholine, a neurotransmitter that is associated with memory. Dr. Benton also found that giving 50 mg/day of thiamine (versus a placebo) was associated with reports of being more clearheaded, composed and energetic.

Now, here's a remarkable fact. The people who reported these wonderful improvements after taking extra thiamine weren't low in thiamine at the start of the study, according to traditional criteria. If you go by the RDA (Recommended Dietary Allowance), their thiamine status was just fine!

Dr. Benton notes that: "Traditionally, the RDA has aimed to avoid a deficiency disease and has added a safety margin. My findings suggest that if you wish to redefine the RDA as achieving optimal functioning then the levels recommended would have to be increased."

And in a direct connection to Alzheimer's, Professor Michael Gold discovered that people with Alzheimer's have lower thiamine levels than those with other types of dementia.

A recommended B1 dosage is 50 – 75 mg.

Vitamin B6 Produces the Chemical Messengers of the Brain

Vitamin B6, or pyridoxine, keeps your blood sugar in normal range. It helps to make hemoglobin, which carries oxygen in red blood cells to your tissues. And it also works to maintain normal nerve function and produce disease-fighting antibodies.

And vitamin B6 plays a key role in the manufacture of neurotransmitters, including serotonin, dopamine, noradrenaline, and adrenaline. These chemicals are your brain's messenger service, allowing thoughts and information to jump from one neuron to the next.

The Mayo Clinic notes that mild deficiency of vitamin B6 is common, and that "Taking pyridoxine supplements in combination with other B vitamins (folic acid and vitamin B12) has been shown to be effective for lowering homocysteine levels."

A recommended dose is 50 - 85 mg. Dr. Marwan Sabbagh in his book, *The Alzheimer's Answer*, writes, "Exceeding 100 mg is not a good idea, since it can cause nerve damage in the feet (peripheral neuropathy).

Vitamin B3 May Cure Alzheimer's for Pennies A Day

Vitamin B3, also known as niacinamide, increases blood flow, lowers cholesterol and plays a key role in energy production.

And now, researchers at University of California Irvine have discovered that niacinamide may be a breakthrough cure for Alzheimer's. In November 2008, a research team headed by Dr. Kim Green published an article in *The Journal of Neuroscience* that described their study of mice genetically engineered to develop Alzheimer's.

For four months, the mice were given daily doses of niacinamide, an easy-to-absorb form of Vitamin B3. At the end of the study, the mice with Alzheimer's tested as well on memory tests as healthy mice.

"**Cognitively, they were cured**," Dr. Green said. "**They performed as if they'd never developed the disease.**" "The vitamin completely prevented cognitive decline associated with the disease, bringing them back to the level they'd be at if they didn't have the pathology."

The scientists observed that niacinamide removed the tell-tale tau protein from the mice's brains. According to Dr. Green, "It's absolutely dramatic." The tau protein "is just wiped from the brain specifically."

The mice were given a high dose of 200 mg/kg per day. Dr. Green's research team is now conducting a human study, in which patients will take 1,500 mg of niacinamide twice daily.

"From my perspective, that's a very tolerable dose of a very inexpensive vitamin. I have been waiting patiently for a break in Alzheimer's disease like this," wrote Dr. Robert Rowen, a pioneering physician who edits *Second Opinion* newsletter.

Taking such high doses of niacinamide is certainly unconventional. But maybe, conventional thinking is wrong.

The Rush Institute for Healthy Aging in Chicago conducted a five-year study of more than 3,700 subjects over age 65, examining their intake of niacin and cognitive function.

Dr. Martha C. Morris, the study's lead author, announced that when subjects with the highest niacin intake were compared to those with the lowest intake, the high niacin group had an *80 percent reduction in risk of developing Alzheimer's* and other forms of cognitive decline.

And when we look at the study's results, once again, we confront the issue of conventional wisdom aiming too low in recommended amounts. The current Recommended Dietary Allowance for niacin is 16 mg per day for men and 14 mg per day for women. And yet, in this study, the group getting a median 14 mg of niacin daily from diet and supplements were at highest risk of developing Alzheimer's.

While some benefits were noted to begin at 17 mg per day, a daily niacin intake of 45 mg offered the most protection from Alzheimer's disease and other causes of cognitive decline.

So what should your dosage of niacinamide be? Many nutritionally minded doctors would recommend a robust daily dose of 50 mg.

But someday in the near future, that amount could go way up. Today's cutting-edge research may discover that taking much higher doses allows people with Alzheimer's to experience the same miracle cure enjoyed by mice.

Whatever your dose, make sure that you take the niacinamide form of B3, as regular niacin can cause marked flushing.

Vitamin C and Vitamin E, the Dynamic Duo for Your Brain

If you want powerful friends in high places – specifically, in your brain - take vitamin C and vitamin E.

Each one offers terrific brain-boosting powers, but taken together, they act like Fred Astaire and Ginger Rogers, dancing in a magical chemistry that no one quite understands yet.

Of course, you already know that vitamin C, or ascorbic acid, famously strengthens the immune system. It's probably the most popular supplement in the world today, since millions use it to fight off colds and other infections and support good health.

But vitamin C can also work wonders in your brain. If you're healthy, you've got lots of vitamin C floating in the fluid that surrounds your brain neurons. There, it serves as a brawny anti-oxidant, capable of delivering knockout blows to free radicals before they damage your brain cells.

A well-known study directly linked vitamin C to intelligence. Schoolchildren from kindergarten to college increased their IQ by an average of nearly 4 points, when they raised their vitamin C intake by 50%.

And in 1997, researchers at Memorial Sloan-Kettering Cancer Center in New York made a big discovery: *vitamin C can readily cross the blood-brain barrier*, when it's traveling in oxidized form.

And now, there's a brand-new study published in the *Journal of Biological Chemistry* that reveals **Vitamin C can dissolve the toxic brain plaque that characterizes Alzheimer's**.

People with Alzheimer's have sticky amyloid plaques in their brain, made of toxic protein clumps. These amyloid plaques eventually kill brain cells, starting in the hippocampus where memory is stored.

"When we treated brain tissue from mice suffering from Alzheimer's disease with vitamin C, we could see that the toxic protein aggregates were dissolved. Our results show a previously unknown model for how Vitamin C affects the amyloid plaques," said Katrin Mani, a researcher in Molecular Medicine at Lund University in Sweden.

"The notion that Vitamin C can have a positive effect on Alzheimer's disease is controversial, but our results open up new opportunities for research into Alzheimer's and the possibilities offered by Vitamin C," said Katrin Mani.

Vitamin E is no slouch, either, in the brain-friendly department. It's a potent antioxidant that dissolves in fat. Since the brain is over 60 percent fat, vitamin E turns out to be enormously useful. It can dissolve inside fatty brain cell membranes, and, once inside, perform sentry duty against free radicals.

And several important studies bear out vitamin E's role in preventing and halting Alzheimer's. Martha C. Morris, Sc.D., the lead nutrition researcher for CHAP, the Chicago Health and Aging Project, monitored vitamin E intake in adults over 65. *Those who took the most Vitamin E were 67 percent less likely to develop Alzheimer's*, compared to the people who took the least. And, the functional difference between these two groups was nothing short of astonishing. Big consumers of vitamin E tested at a mental level <u>8 to 10 years younger</u> than people taking low amounts.

CHAP researchers also discovered that if people did develop Alzheimer's, they declined at a noticeably slower rate, providing they consumed enough vitamin E.

Other researchers have confirmed these findings. Dr. Alireza Atri at Massachusetts General Hospital (MGH), the VA Bedford Medical Center, and Harvard Medical School, Boston, led a study of 540 patients with Alzheimer's who were being treated at the MGH Memory Disorders Units.

In 2009, Dr. Atri's group reported that patients who were given high doses of vitamin E (from 800 units daily to 1000 units twice daily), fared noticeably better in their ability to carry out personal tasks like getting dressed than other groups being tested, over a three-year period.

And let's not leave out the famous Baltimore Longitudinal Study of Aging. Researchers at Johns Hopkins honed in on the data of 579 older participants in the study. And they discovered that, over a nine-month period, the big consumers of vitamin E had the least chance of getting Alzheimer's.

Dr. David Perlmutter, a board-certified neurologist and leading expert on the brain, wrote, "taking vitamin E can buy you a decade's worth of brain power. That's why I think that *everyone* should take this powerful antioxidant every day."

Now that you're excited about what vitamin C and vitamin E can do on their own, consider the sensational results when they join together. We'll zoom from Honolulu to Utah to Holland, checking out some significant studies.

HONOLULU: 3,400 older Japanese-American men took supplements of vitamin C and vitamin E at least once a week. Analysis from the Honolulu Aging Study found they were **88 per cent less likely to develop vascular dementia** than those who didn't! After Alzheimer's, vascular is the most common form of dementia.

UTAH: 4,740 elderly residents of Cache County, Utah had their medical records analyzed by researchers from The Johns Hopkins University Bloomberg School of Public Health in Baltimore. The researchers found the greatest reduction of Alzheimer's in participants who used individual vitamin E and C supplements in combination, with or without an additional multivitamin.

"Use of vitamin E and C (ascorbic acid) supplements in combination reduced AD [Alzheimer's disease] prevalence [by about 78 percent] and incidence [by about 64 percent]," wrote the researchers.

Once again, we encounter the issue that the RDA (Recommended Dietary Allowance) may not be nearly enough to get the job done.

"The current… recommended daily allowance for vitamin E is 22 IU (15 micrograms), and for vitamin C (ascorbic acid), 75 to 90 micrograms," the researchers wrote. "Multivitamin preparations typically contain these approximate quantities of both vitamins E and C (more vitamin C in some instances), while individual supplements typically contain doses up to 1,000 IU of vitamin E and 500 to 1,000 micrograms or more of vitamin C (ascorbic acid). Our findings suggest that vitamins E and C may offer protection against AD when taken together in the higher doses available from individual supplements."

HOLLAND: 5,500 people aged 55 and older were tracked over six years in Holland. Those who took high doses of vitamins C and E lessened their risk of Alzheimer's by 18 percent, regardless of age, gender, smoking, weight and education. Smokers got the biggest benefit.

So what dosage should you take? As you can see in the Utah study above, controversy reigns about optimal amounts for both vitamin C and vitamin E.

Dr. Jacob Teitelbaum suggests:

• **Vitamin C (500-1,000 mg/day)**

• **Vitamin E (100 units/day)**

Dr. Teitelbaum says of vitamin E, "This critical antioxidant serves many functions, but more is not always better. Many nutrients (such as beta carotene) are part of a larger "family," so taking very high doses of only one type can actually suppress the others and become problematic. This is the case with vitamin E as well, as there are many types of tocopherols. Research suggests that taking over 150 units a day can actually be problematic, so I recommend taking 100 units a day as the optimal level in multi-vitamins. If you are taking higher levels to treat a specific problem, take it for only a few months and use natural vitamin E (mixed tocopherols) which contain all of the different types of vitamin E."

So which type of vitamin E should you take? The answer is surprisingly complicated, but if you get it right, the health benefits can be immense.

Here's how the *Cancer Defeated* newsletter explains the problem: "For starters, there are actually *eight* types of vitamin E. Four are **"tocopherols,"** and four are **"tocotrienols."** Each group has an alpha, beta, gamma, and delta subtype. The main difference between tocopherols and tocotrienols is a slight variation in chemical structure."

"When you buy vitamin E supplements in the store, chances are you're buying alpha-tocopherol. The ingredient list might say "alpha-tocopherol and mixed tocopherols," but the reality is that it's mostly alpha-tocopherol. Few vitamin E supplements include any form of tocotrienols."

"Yet by some estimates, tocotrienols are 50 times more powerful than tocopherols. This makes them much more effective in disease prevention. Of course, they're also a lot more expensive. But for those who can afford it, the benefits are extreme."

Lee Euler of *Cancer Defeated* explains that the scientific community is now paying more attention to tocotrienols. In the past few years, almost 30% of the peer-reviewed studies on vitamin E have been specific to tocotrienols, rising from less than 1% in previous years.

So far, studies indicate that tocotrienols are safe. They appear to have no adverse effects when taken for a period as long as four years (the length of the longest study to date).

But the controversy over the right dosages of vitamins C and E continues to rage.

Here's what Dr. David Perlmutter recommends for people with serious cognitive issues:

• **Vitamin C: 200 mgs twice daily for a total of 400 mg daily**

• **Vitamin E: 400 IU daily** (buy d-alpha tocopherol and NOT di-alpha tocopherol)

• **Dr. Perlmutter recommends that Alzheimer's patients take a higher dosage of vitamin C: 500 mg in the morning and 500 mg at night**

And Dr. Ronald Hoffman describes his regimen for an Alzheimer's patient on his website.

• **Vitamin C: 4 gms (4,000 mgs) daily**

• **Vitamin E: 800 IU daily**

Since the recommendations for Vitamin C and E vary widely, you should talk with your doctor about the right amount of supplementation for you.

Vitamin D Is the Sunshine of Your Life

The controversies that swirl around vitamin D are loud, passionate, and tremendously urgent. Let's start with the frightening fact that over 33% of older adults are so lacking in Vitamin D that they're putting their lives at risk.

"It's likely that more than one-third of older adults now have vitamin D levels associated with higher risks of death and few have levels associated with optimum survival," said Adit Ginde, MD, MPH, an assistant professor at the University of Colorado Denver School of Medicine's Division of Emergency Medicine. Dr. Ginde, the lead author of a study published in 2009, evaluated the link between Vitamin D levels and death rates in people 65 and older.

One big reason that millions of people lack vitamin D is that they're scared to expose themselves to sun. For years, doctors have shouted from the rooftops about the dangers of sunlight. And since 90% of our vitamin D comes from exposure to sun, enormous numbers of people aren't getting even the minimal amounts of sunshine they need.

Dr. Jacob Teitelbaum has strong feelings on the subject. He says that multiple studies have shown that Vitamin D deficiencies can cause cancer. And, tragically, the medical establishment's misguided advice on avoiding sun has led thousands of cancer victims to lose their lives from insufficient Vitamin D.

I'll let Dr. Teitelbaum tell you a bit about how the controversy plays out in the academic world:

"Of course, having scientific research behind you may not offer much protection in academia," writes Dr. Teitelbaum. "One of the world's leading experts on vitamin D is Dr. Michael Holick, chief of endocrinology, nutrition and diabetes (and in the past a professor of dermatology) at Boston University. He published a book, *The UV Advantage*, urging people to get enough sunlight to make vitamin D. "I am advocating common sense, not prolonged sunbathing or tanning salons," Holick said.

"Repeated sunburns especially in childhood and among redheads and very fair-skinned people have been linked to melanoma, but there is no credible scientific evidence that moderate sun exposure causes it," Holick contends. "The problem has been that the American Academy of Dermatology has been unchallenged for 20 years," he says. "They have brainwashed the public at every level." Despite the strong evidence supporting the role of common sense (i.e., avoid sunburn, not sunshine), the head of Holick's department, Dr. Barbara Gilchrest, called his book an embarrassment and stripped him of his dermatology professorship."

As you get older, you ratchet up additional risk factors for low vitamin D. Your ability to process it declines, and you're more likely to be housebound in the hazardous winter months.

And that brings us to the growing link between vitamin D deficiencies and dementia. A recent study published in *Archives of Internal Medicine* investigated 858 adults aged 65 and older, over a six-year period. The subjects with lowest vitamin D levels -- less than 25 nanomoles per liter of blood -- were 60% more likely to exhibit signs of general cognitive decline. And they were 31% more likely to suffer deteriorated executive function – the ability to plan, organize, and prioritize.

"Our study demonstrates that low levels of vitamin D are associated with an increased risk of new cognitive problems," said study researcher David J. Llewellyn, PhD, of the University of Exeter, England.

Some intriguing lab research published in 2011 suggests that vitamin D helps to remove amyloid-beta protein, which forms the sticky brain plaques that characterize Alzheimer's.

Researchers from Tohoku University, Japan discovered that vitamin D injections improved the removal of amyloid from the brain of mice.

Professor Tetsuya Terasaki said, "Vitamin D appears to increase transport of amyloid β across the blood brain barrier (BBB) by regulating protein expression, via the vitamin D receptor, and also by regulating cell signaling via the MEK pathway. These results lead the way towards new therapeutic targets in the search for prevention of Alzheimer's disease."

I spoke to Dr. Tara Peyman, a naturopathic physician in Arizona, about vitamin D, and asked her if she can recommend a particular brand.

"I like Pure Encapsulations," said Dr. Peyman. "It's easy and affordable. It's in the form of liquid drops. Some of the liquids go bad easily, and this one doesn't seem to."

"Vitamin D is fat soluble, so you need to take it with oil. If you take it in powder or tablet form, it won't absorb well, unless you take it with fish oil or some other oil. But Pure Encapsulations is emulsified in oil, so you don't need to worry about that. I usually recommend 10,000 IU for people who are very deficient, but that should be determined with a doctor."

Here's what the Pure Encapsulations website says about their product:

"Pure Encapsulations Vitamin D_3 liquid provides 1,000 i.u. per drop, an ideal daily amount. For individuals with greater short-term needs, this product allows for achieving 25,000-50,000 i.u. vitamin D_3 per week without having to take multiple capsules. For the elderly, Vitamin D_3 liquid is an easy to use form. Vitamin D_3 liquid, in a base of medium chain triglycerides, does not require emulsification for absorption. Vitamin D_3 liquid is also free of preservatives, artificial colors, flavors and sugars."

How much Vitamin D people with cognitive difficulties should take is another controversy. Recommendations range from 400 IU to 5,000 IU, or even 10,000, in extreme cases. Dr. Holick's book, *The UV Advantage*, is a good source of information on this controversy and on how to determine the proper dose for you with the help of a doctor and a blood test.

If you're unable to afford a doctor consultation, it's good to know that very few people, if any, will be endangered by supplementing with 2000 IU per day. Most of us can benefit from significantly more, but that's where a doctor's advice is needed. It's very important to take D3, not the less effective D2. The type of vitamin D needed to enrich milk – D2 – is much less effective.

Sources:

Dr. Jacob Teitelbaum's website:
www.endfatigue.com

Pure Encapsulations Vitamin D3
http://pureencapsulations.com/

Ray Sahelian
www.raysahelian.com/alzheimer.html

Daily Mail
"10p pill to beat Alzheimer's disease: Vitamin B halts memory loss in breakthrough British trial"
Fiona MacRae
September 9, 2010
http://www.dailymail.co.uk/health/article-1310330/Vitamin-B-halts-memory-loss-10p-pill-beat-Alzheimers-disease.html#ixzz1i2u0l562

The Healthier Life
"Niacin Found to Reduce the Risk of Cognitive Decline"
June 1, 2006
http://www.thehealthierlife.co.uk/natural-health-articles/alzheimers/niacin-reduce-risk-cognitive-decline-00019.html

Lancet
"Effect of 3-year folic acid supplementation on cognitive function in older adults in the FACIT trial: a randomised, double blind, controlled trial."
Durga J, van Boxtel MP, Schouten EG, Kok FJ, Jolles J, Katan MB, Verhoef P
2007 Jan 20;369(9557):208-16.
www.ncbi.nlm.nih.gov/pubmed/17240287

Science Daily
"Treatment with Vitamin C Dissolves Protein Aggregates in Alzheimer's Disease"
August 18, 2011
www.sciencedaily.com/releases/2011/08/110818101645.htm

Cache County, Utah Study:
JAMA and Archives Journal
"Using vitamin E and C supplements together may reduce risk of Alzheimer disease"
January 19, 2004
www.eurekalert.org/pub_releases/2004-01/jaaj-uve011404.php

Honolulu Aging Study
Neurology 2000 Mar 28;54(6):1265-72.
"Association of vitamin E and C supplement use with cognitive function and dementia in elderly men."
Masaki KH, Losonczy KG, Izmirlian G, Foley DJ, Ross GW, Petrovitch H, Havlik R,

White LR
http://www.ncbi.nlm.nih.gov/pubmed/10746596

Holland Study
JAMA June 26, 2002
"Dietary intake of antioxidants and risk of Alzheimer disease."
Engelhart MJ, Geerlings MI, Ruitenberg A, van Swieten JC, Hofman A, Witteman JC, Breteler MM
http://www.ncbi.nlm.nih.gov/pubmed/12076218

Web MD
"Vitamins D and E May Affect Dementia Risk"
Denise Mann
July 12, 2010
http://www.webmd.com/brain/news/20100712/vitamins-d-and-e-may-affect-dementia-risk

"Fluids and Barriers of the CNS"
"1α,25-Dihydroxyvitamin D_3 enhances cerebral clearance of human amyloid-β peptide(1-40) from mouse brain across the blood-brain barrier"
Shingo Ito, Sumio Ohtsuki, Yasuko Nezu, Yusuke Koitabashi, Sho Murata and Tetsuya Terasaki
July 8, 2011
www.fluidsbarrierscns.com/content/8/1/20

Science Daily
"Advances in Research in Alzheimer's Disease"
July 9, 2011
http://www.sciencedaily.com/releases/2011/07/110709113610.htm

The Telegraph
"Supplements of Vitamin D could cut Alzheimer's Risk"
by Chris Irvine
January 23, 2009
http://www.telegraph.co.uk/health/elderhealth/4319390/Supplements-of-vitamin-D-could-cut-Alzheimers-risk.html

Cancer Defeated
"Eight Types of Vitamin E – And the Most Popular One is the WRONG One!"
By Lee Euler
Issue 138
http://cancerdefeatedpublications.com/newsletters/The-WRONG-kind-of-vitamin-E.html

The World's Healthiest Foods
Vitamin E
http://www.whfoods.com/genpage.php?tname=nutrient&dbid=111

Science Daily
"Insufficient Levels Of Vitamin D Puts Elderly At Increased Risk Of Dying From Heart Disease"
Sep. 21, 2009
www.sciencedaily.com/releases/2009/09/090921134654.htm

Natural Health Archives
"Will This Remarkably Inexpensive Nutrient Cure Alzheimer's Disease"
Dr. Robert Rowen, M.D.
http://www.naturalhealtharchives.com/alzheimer's-disease-niacinamide-vitamin-B3.php

The Journal of Clinical Investigation:
Published in Volume 100, Issue 11 (December 1, 1997)
J Clin Invest. 1997;100(11):2842–2848. doi:10.1172/JCI119832.
Copyright © 1997, The American Society for Clinical Investigation.
Research Article
"Vitamin C crosses the blood-brain barrier in the oxidized form through the glucose transporters."
D B Agus, S S Gambhir, W M Pardridge, C Spielholz, J Baselga, J C Vera and D W Golde
Memorial Sloan-Kettering Cancer Center, New York, New York 10021, USA. d-agus@ski.mskcc.org
Published December 1, 1997
www.jci.org/articles/view/119832

The Better Brain Book
David Perlmutter, M.D., FACN and Carol Colman
Riverhead Books, 2004

The Anti-Alzheimer's Prescription
Vincent Fortanasce, M.D.
Gotham Books, 2008

The Alzheimer's Answer
Marwan Sabbagh, M.D.
John Wiley & Sons, 2008

The Alzheimer's Prevention Plan

Patrick Holford with Shane Heaton and Deborah Colson

Piatkus Books, 2005

The Inflammation Syndrome

Jack Challem

John Wiley & Sons, 2010

Chapter 18

Mangosteen Revives Dad Like "A Watered Plant"

One day, while trolling the Internet for more juicy facts about Alzheimer's remedies, I came upon a startling story. Coleen Melsted had posted this testimonial in an Alzheimer's chat room:

My Father at the young age of 64 started having problems at work and had to retire early. He was then diagnosed with a very aggressive form of Alzheimer's. He is now in a home because my mother couldn't handle him anymore. He worked as a very successful Autobodyman and may have ingested a lot of chemicals. A friend of mine gave me a bottle of [mangosteen juice] and I had read that it may help with Alzheimer's. We thought we would have nothing to lose as he is now in a very vegetative state. He didn't know anyone, he couldn't feed himself and he couldn't even talk anymore.

We got him on 1 oz of [mangosteen juice] per day and on the 5th day he called my son by his name. We were all shocked! He continued taking 1 oz per day and he has now been feeding himself consistently for 25 days!

He is more alert and happy. He even looks and smiles at me when I visit him. He is now even communicating with us a little. We are now increasing his dosage to 2 oz per day with his doctors' blessing and we are all excited to see what happens.

This product has created much excitement for our family! I wish we would have had this product 5 years ago. I want people to understand that my father is pretty far gone but has had somewhat amazing results due to taking this product. I truly believe this product offers new hope to other people...

Coleen Melsted

Update: Hi Everyone this testimonial really needs an update. My dad is doing great. He's walking, talking, eating on his own, happy, very familiar with family members and friends! He's improving everyday! We are all very excited to see where he will be in the next few months. This has really added quality to his life and ours as well. I encourage you to let people know about this juice, you may be able to help them avoid what our family has gone through!

Have a great day!

Coleen

Well, that certainly sounded interesting! After some sleuthing, I managed to track down Coleen's phone number, and reached her at her home in Canada on my very first try.

Coleen was eager to talk about mangosteen juice, and tell me more about her father's stunning transformation. "My father had a very aggressive form of Alzheimer's and was deteriorating really fast," Coleen explained. "He was down to a vegetable in a chair. Somebody gave me a bottle of the juice and I gave it to my mom and said it's worth a try."

"Well, my mom called me and said, 'You've got to come see this! It's like somebody watered the plant and he came back to life!' My dad was lively, talking to other people, enjoying himself, walking around."

I asked Coleen how quickly her father responded to the mangosteen juice.

"He reacted within the first five days," she said. "People who are ill react faster. When I went on mangosteen juice myself, it took about three and a half months for me to realize that my environmental allergies and joint pain from synchronized skating were gone. You get used to living with those things and don't pay attention."

"My father had been told that he had 18 months to live. Well, he lived another seven and a half years! It was unbelievable. My mom's skeptical about this stuff, but she saw that he went from no communication to being up and around and taking care of himself."

"When my friends heard about it, they began asking me, do you think mangosteen juice will help with my diabetes…or my tendonitis? They asked if I'd sell them my bottles of it, and I said, 'No! I need them for my dad!' "

"So, after a while, I began selling mangosteen juice and now I'm a distributor. I just wish my dad had taken it earlier. He wouldn't have had to go into care."

After talking to Coleen, I was determined to learn more. Quickly, I found myself plunged into the exotic world of the mangosteen.

The Queen of Fruits Brims with Antioxidant Xanthones

It's not a mango. It's an Asian tropical fruit, mostly cultivated in Thailand, that's so beloved it's called the Queen of Fruits. In 1930, botanist David Fairchild described the mangosteen with these mouthwatering words: ''It is so delicate that it melts in the mouth like ice cream. The flavor is quite indescribably delicious. There is nothing to mar the perfection of this fruit…''

More recently, *The New York Times* lauded the mangosteen as "a tropical fruit about the size of a tangerine, whose leathery maroon shell surrounds moist, fragrant, snow-white segments of ambrosial flesh…"

I've yet to eat a mangosteen, but after reading that, I'm ready to get on a plane to Thailand! But however tasty the mangosteen's inner fruit may be, the source of its health-giving powers lies within its thick rind and seeds.

The mangosteen's rind, also known as the pericarp, brims with **xanthones**, a little-known type of antioxidant that packs a powerful punch. Xanthones hunt down free radicals and show them no mercy. And mounting clinical evidence indicates that xanthones successfully reduce inflammation, a crucial asset for treating inflamed Alzheimer's brains.

Are there reams of studies on mangosteen's effect on Alzheimer's patients? Frankly, no, at least not that I could find.

The evidence for mangosteen on Alzheimer's patients is anecdotal. But it's also backed up by a growing stack of clinical data, analyzing mangosteen's xanthones and phytonutrients in the lab.

My search of the National Institutes of Health database yielded 156 entries on mangosteen. Here's a sample taste of recent studies with strong relevance for Alzheimer's. One study examined xanthones' protection of brain tissue. Another investigated its antioxidant impact.

Brain tissue protection

The natural xanthone alpha-mangostin reduces oxidative damage in rat brain tissue. *Nutr Neurosci.* 2009. Laboratorio de Aminoácidos Excitadores, Instituto Nacional de Neurología y Neurocirugía Manuel Velasco Suárez, Insurgentes Sur México DF, Mexico.

The antiperoxidative properties of alpha-mangostin, a xanthone isolated from mangosteen fruit, were tested for the first time in nerve tissue exposed to different toxic insults. Two reliable biological preparations (rat brain homogenates and synaptosomal P2 fractions) were exposed to the toxic actions of a free radical generator (ferrous sulfate), an excitotoxic agent (quinolinate), and a mitochondrial toxin (3-nitropropionate). Alpha-mangostin decreased the lipoperoxidative action of FeSO(4) in both preparations in a concentration-dependent manner, and completely abolished the peroxidative effects of quinolinate, 3-nitropropionate and FeSO(4) + quinolinate at all concentrations tested. Interestingly, when tested alone in brain homogenates, alpha-mangostin significantly decreased the lipoperoxidation even below basal levels. Alpha-mangostin exerts a robust antiperoxidative effect in brain tissue preparations probably through its properties as a free radical scavenger. In light of these findings, this antioxidant should be tested in other neurotoxic models involving oxidative stress.

Antioxidant benefit

Bioavailability and antioxidant effects of a xanthone-rich Mangosteen (Garcinia mangostana) product in humans.

J Agric Food Chem. 2009. Brunswick Laboratories, Norton, Massachusetts, USA. This study investigated the absorption and antioxidant effects of a xanthone-rich mangosteen liquid in healthy human volunteers after the acute consumption of 59 mL of the supplement. The liquid contained mangosteen, aloe vera, green tea, and multivitamins. Results indicated that alpha-mangostin and vitamins B(2) and B(5) were bioavailable. The antioxidant capacity measured with the oxygen radical absorbance capacity (ORAC) assay was increased with a maximum effect of 18% after 2 hours, and the increased antioxidant level lasted at least 4 hours. Overall, this study demonstrated the bioavailability of antioxidants from a xanthone-rich mangosteen product and its in vivo antioxidant effects.

"The Most Powerful Anti-Inflammatory I've Seen in 30 Years of Practice"

Dr. Kenneth J. Finsand, a chiropractic physician and the author of *The Mangosteen Desk Reference*, says, "This is probably the most famous use of all the qualities found in the mangosteen: **it is by far the most powerful anti-inflammatory I have ever seen in 30 years of practice.** Research has proven this to be true, along with folk medicine history."

Dr. Finsand has personal reason to champion mangosteen. In 1981, he suffered a devastating back injury while surfing. Over the years, the chronic pain worsened, and he felt exhausted and sick, possibly due to his long-term use of medication.

In 2002, Dr. Finsand discovered mangosteen juice and experienced a dramatic recovery of his health.

"Because of the amazing results I have had with mangosteen, I am now drug-free and virtually pain-free for the first time in 21 years. The research I have performed on this product has led me to believe that it helps restore liver function, it breaks down insulin resistance, and it can turn around chronic conditions of inflammation in the cells of the body."

"Amazing" Renewal for Alzheimer's Patients in Adult Care Home!

The more I read about mangosteen, the more fascinated I became. And then, I discovered this story on a website dedicated to testimonials about a mangosteen juice product:

"My name is Barbara G. I am General Manager of an adult care home in Arizona. A few months ago, one of our residents' daughters brought a bottle of mangosteen juice to our adult care home to try on her mother who has Alzheimer's disease. This resident is 86 years old.

The results were amazing. Prior to taking mangosteen juice, she was sleeping most of the day and it was very difficult to carry on a conversation with her. Now, after taking mangosteen juice for approximately three months, she is alert during the day, vibrant and easy to communicate with. Since her results were so exciting, we began giving mangosteen juice to four of our other residents with outstanding results.

Resident 1 is a 72 year old Alzheimer's patient who prior to taking mangosteen juice was sleeping all day, would not communicate and could not feed herself. Now after two months on mangosteen juice, she does not sleep all day, she is alert, communicates with others and feeds herself.

Resident 2 is an 86 year old Alzheimer's patient, is blind, has very stiff muscles, she has not talked or opened her eyes for several years and is bed bound. After being on mangosteen juice for approximately two months, she now talks at times, moves her arms and legs occasionally and communicates without screaming. She now opens her eyes and is aware of her surroundings.

Resident 3 is a 76 year old who has Parkinson's disease. Prior to taking mangosteen juice she was very quiet, stayed in her room all day. Now after two months on mangosteen juice, she comes out of her room for meals, is a lot stronger, her appetite has increased, and she now walks with minimal assistance.

Resident 4 is a 94 year old who is very frail, has transfusions every three months, has a poor appetite and is anemic. Now, after being on mangosteen juice for almost two months, she is eating well, much stronger and very happy.

After seeing the wonderful results that the residents were experiencing, I started taking mangosteen juice myself. I was suffering from migraine headaches. I have now gone several months with no migraine headaches. When I begin to feel the symptoms of a migraine, I double up on the mangosteen juice dosage and do not have migraines. My energy level has also increased since being on mangosteen juice.

I am also giving mangosteen juice to my nine year old son who suffers from asthma and sinus infections year round. After taking mangosteen juice his asthma medications have been decreased. When a sinus infection flares up, I double the dosage of mangosteen juice and his sinus infection is gone in two to three days. Also, my four year old niece had no appetite, would vomit at the sight of food, was very skinny and pale. She has been on mangosteen juice for several months. She is now eating very well, has gained weight, has rosy cheeks and less sinus infections. Mangosteen juice has truly been a miracle in a short period of time for my family and for the residents at the facility I manage."

Well, Barbara's story certainly sounds encouraging.

Which Mangosteen Juice Product Is Right for You?

Unfortunately, you can't get the xanthones you need by eating lots of delicious mangosteen fruit every day. It's still very difficult to find mangosteen in the United States, because the government restricts its import for fear of pests. And the mangosteen tree needs humid, tropical climates and can't be grown anywhere in the U.S.

Even if you ate the fruit, you still wouldn't receive the real healing power of mangosteen, because the rind and seeds contain most of the xanthones. You must consume them, too, to get mangosteen's full therapeutic impact.

In 2002, six partners formed a company they dubbed Xango, a name derived from XAN for xanthones and GO from mangosteen. And they set about creating the first mangosteen juice product on the market. Xango Juice uses the whole fruit, including the rind, seed and pulp. And to compensate for the rind's less-than-sweet flavor, Xango's makers added a variety of other juices to improve the taste.

You can't go to the grocery and buy Xango. It's sold by individual distributors, including Coleen Melsted, whose story you heard at the beginning of this chapter. However, you can buy it online, along with various other mangosteen-derived products that Xango now makes, in addition to its juice product.

In the wake of Xango's success, other companies chimed in with a mangosteen fruit juice of their own. Here's where things get tricky. A mangosteen juice product may sound better, because it's 100% mangosteen juice and doesn't contain other juices that dilute it.

However, if it's 100% mangosteen juice, it may only contain the fleshy part of the fruit. It probably doesn't include the whole rind, which contains most of the xanthones and other important phytonutrients.

So a 100% mangosteen fruit juice may sound better and even taste better, and yet, not provide the full scope of healing nourishment that you're seeking.

According to Xango, "At this point in time, we are the only company to use the entire mangosteen fruit, including the nutrient-rich rind known as the pericarp, in a beverage."

An alternative to juice might be a mangosteen extract pill, which contains both the fruit and rind. Dr. Ray Sahelian is a physician and nutrition expert who frequently writes about natural supplements. He also formulates his own line of supplements, which you can obtain through his website – www.raysahelian.com.

Dr. Sahelian produces a mangosteen pill, and here's what he says about it:

Mangosteen pill 500 mg (whole fruit and rind) - direct from Thailand
Developed by Ray Sahelian, M.D.
Made from the highest quality ORGANIC raw material available, direct from Thailand. The actual active ingredients, xanthones, are mostly in the rind and seed, and less in the fruit. We use the whole fruit - rind, seed and fruit - in order to provide you with the full spectrum of xanthones. There are about 20 different xanthones in the whole fruit. Half of this product is rind, the other half whole fruit.

Supplement facts
Mangosteen 500 mg (Garcinia mangostana whole fruit and pericarp or rind)

I certainly can't claim that mangosteen is a guaranteed miracle worker for Alzheimer's. But on the other hand, there are no known contraindications with mangosteen fruit juice and medications.

So you might want to try drinking a refreshing ounce or two in the morning, and see what happens. Here's to your health!

Sources:

Xango
www.xango.com

Ray Sahelian
www.raysahelian.com
www.raysahelian.com/xanthones.html

My Mangosteen (distributor)
www.onlinemangosteen.com

Mangosteen Research
www.researchmangosteen.com

Xango Testimonials
Alzheimer's, Parkinson's Disease, Migraine
September 4, 2004
www.xangotestimonials.blogspot.com
http://www.mangosteeneffect.com/testimonial-detail.php?id=13

Mangosteen and Health: Alzheimer's Disease
www.mangosteen-juice-online.com/mangosteen-health-alzheimers-disease.html

MangosteenTree.ca
Dr. Kenneth J. Finsand
http://mangosteentree.ca/medical/drfinsand.html

Chapter 19

Taking Your Next Step

You've just learned a lot about Alzheimer's, and you may be wondering how to start using this new information. Perhaps it all seems a bit overwhelming.

My suggestion is that you begin by taking heart. You have more roads to healing than you realized, and a world of new possibilities lies before you.

Your first step may be to find a doctor who's sympathetic to these approaches and is willing to work with you. Your current doctor may fit the bill, or you may need to reach out to other physicians who are more open-minded and flexible.

Get the Right Tests to Get the Right Diagnosis

Make sure you get tested to eliminate other causes of cognitive decline. As you learned in the preceding chapters, nutritional deficits can provoke brain dysfunction. So can a host of other overlooked problems, including depression, thyroid problems, chronic infections, and excess medications.

You may want to take a free, 15-minute online test that will give you instant feedback about your cognitive state. The Cognitive Function Test was devised by scientists at Oxford University and can be taken in the comfort of your own home. You'll work your way through three sections using computer-based games to test different components of your memory. You can take The Cognitive Function Test at **www.foodforthebrain.org**.

Good Nutrition for A Healthier Brain

Fill your plate with lots of lean proteins and fresh vegetables, along with smaller helpings of fruit and whole grains, seeds, and nuts. Push away the sugary, starchy, processed foods and sodas.

And choose a supplement described here and start taking it. Make notes about how you're doing. Then try taking something else, and something else again. Experiment with different doses and combinations.

Your Journey to Renewed Mental Clarity and Vigor

Stay encouraged. Stay positive. Stay open to new ideas.

Others have found their way back from Alzheimer's, using the strategies that are detailed here. The next story of reversing Alzheimer's and reclaiming a fulfilling life could be yours.

Here are some sources for additional information that you may find helpful.

Websites:

National Institutes of Health
National Institute on Aging
Alzheimer's Disease Education and Referral Center
Call toll-free:
1-800-438-4380
Mon-Fri, 8:30 am-5:00 pm Eastern Time
or email:
adear@nia.nih.gov
www.nia.nih.gov/alzheimers

Alzheimer's Weekly
www.alzheimersweekly.com

Alzheimer's Association
www.alz.org

Alzheimer's Foundation of America
www.alzfdn.org

Alzheimer's Reading Room
www.alzheimersreadingroom.com

Books:

The Better Brain Book
David Perlmutter, M.D., FACN and Carol Colman
Riverhead Books, 2004

The Anti-Alzheimer's Prescription
Vincent Fortanasce, M.D.
Gotham Books, 2008

The Alzheimer's Answer

Marwan Sabbagh, M.D.

John Wiley & Sons, 2008

The Alzheimer's Prevention Plan

Patrick Holford with Shane Heaton and Deborah Colson

Piatkus Books, 2005

100 Simple Things You Can Do to Prevent Alzheimer's

Jean Carper

Little, Brown and Company, 2010

The Inflammation Syndrome

Jack Challem

John Wiley & Sons, 2010